THE SOCIAL EFFECTS OF HEALTH POLICY

The Social Effects of Health Policy

Experiences of Health and Health Care in Contemporary Britain

JOHN EYLES
McMaster University, Canada
and
JENNY DONOVAN
London Hospital Medical School

Avebury

Aldershot · Brookfield USA · Hong Kong · Singapore · Sydney

Published by
Avebury
Gower Publishing Company Limited
Gower House
Croft Road
Aldershot
Hants   GU11 3HR
England

Gower Publishing Company
Old Post Road
Brookfield
Vermont   05036
USA

Reprinted 1993

IBSN 0 566 07084 7

Contents

Preface

The purpose of this book is to describe how white working class and black people living in the metropolitan areas of England perceive their health and experience the health care system. In this study, we are concerned to show the relationships between health, illness and health care on the one hand, and society in general on the other. Our title though reflects that the experience of social life can be affected by the nature of policy, in this case health policy. Health and illness are grounded and explored in relation to social life in general.

In our study, we have tried to explore the relations between lay perceptions of health and illness on the one hand and health policy and research methodology on the other. We have though tried to moderate our use of jargon and technical discussion so that the book may be accessible to both lay and academic audiences. It has of course been necessary to enter such discussion especially in chapters 2 and 7. Even in these, we place some of the theoretical, policy and methodological material in notes.

In writing this book, many people have been of great assistance. We must acknowledge the financial contribution provided by the Economic and Social Research Council (ESRC). They funded the research project, which is the basis of the studies of the white working class in the three metropolitan areas of Greater London, West Midlands and West Yorkshire. In the text, these are respectively represented by the fictitious names of Parkheath, referred to in the quotations as PH; Moosley Green, as MG; and Deanswood as DW. The ESRC also funded Donovan's research studentship on black people's health which led to her doctorate. Extracts from this study of people of Asian and Afro-Caribbean descent, referred to respectively in quotations by AS and AC, are based on that Ph.D., partly previously published by Gower as 'We don't buy sickness, it just comes' (1986). We should also point out that J. in the text refers to the interviewer.

We must also thank the research secretary at Queen Mary College, Carol Purton, who diligently and good-humouredly transcribed many of the tapes and typed earlier papers and drafts of the project. Pat Kirkpatrick and Shirley Rodway took our handwritten manuscript and turned them rapidly into typescript. Rosanna Wan, at McMaster University under great pressures, transformed the typescript in the polished and professional camera ready copy. We would like to thank her and the Department of Geography at McMaster for allowing the project to draw on its limited resources. A great debt is also owed by us to our families, Dorothy, Pete and David, for their understanding and patience. We dedicate the results of our work to them. But finally and perhaps most importantly, we are indebted to all our respondents without whom there would be no study. As with the places, doctors and institutions, we have changed their names.

                                   John Eyles
                                   Jenny Donovan

                                   Dundas, Ontario
                                   Tottenham, London

1 Health in Britain

INTRODUCTION

This is a book about how working class people, both black and
white, perceive their health and experience the health care
system. But people do not talk about and experience health
and health care in a vacuum. Health is very much part of life
itself. We need good health to work, bring up children and
enjoy life to the full. Poor health is often associated with
incapacity for work, unemployment and stressful and blighted
social and family life. For us, as individuals then, health
is related to other facets of life. We give it an extremely
high priority(1), whether or not it is cause, effect or both
of a satisfying or disadvantaged life.

Health and health care are also part of society in general
and the nature of British society will shape our views on what
is healthy, the characteristics of the health care system and
the possibilities of enjoying a healthy life. A healthy life
does not simply exist. Nor is it a matter of our own making
alone. The economy and the jobs it provides and the housing
market and the quality of accommodation as well as our own
social characteristics - age, gender, ethnicity, social status
- and what these mean in society will influence health.
Because of the importance of this social context for health -
one identified by our study populations themselves as we shall
see in Chapter 4 - we begin this opening chapter by briefly
looking at life in Britain. What is British society like and
how is structured? The answers to these questions allow us
to go on to see how the social structure of Britain is
manifested in health, particularly in inequalities in health
status and health care provision. These inequalities have
been addressed by policy and these will be briefly considered
before we conclude the chapter by demonstrating how the
material in this book raises policy issues as well as informs

1

on working class perceptions of health and health care.

LIFE IN BRITAIN

A broad and generalised view of the post-1945 period in
Britain would conclude that there has been a steady
improvement in living conditions and standards for the vast
majority of the people.(2)   To be sure, the increases in
prosperity have not been as great as those achieved in other
capitalist nations but the increases have been, by and large,
steady and maintained with, it could be argued, due attention
being paid to social welfare needs as well as material
conditions. For the thirty years or so after the Second World
War, most people became progressively wealthier.   Real
personal disposal income per head and real consumer
expenditure per head both increased. Between 1951 and 1977,
for example, average earnings for a man in manual work
increased in real terms by 71 per cent. Not only were people
better off but the earnings differences between manual and
non-manual workers and between men and women were also
narrowing.   Greater prosperity appeared to be married to
greater equality, with respect to type of job and gender.
Income and wealth were also gradually being redistributed.
While this was mainly a redistribution within the wealthiest
half of the British population, some extra resources did
filter down to the poorest households.   This filtering was
assisted by the commitment of various governments to welfare
and the provision of subsidies. The numbers receiving old age
pensions doubled between 1951 and 1978, although at all times
the pension has always been below one half of average male
manual earnings. The range of subsidies was extended to those
in housing need,the disabled and mentally handicapped, amongst
others.(3)   The commitment to welfare was seen in greatly
increased public expenditure which in fact doubled in real
terms between 1961 and 1975.

The prosperity of the vast majority of the British people
was reflected in changing spending and consumption patterns.
Throughout the 1960s and 1970s the proportions spent on food,
clothing and footwear fell, while that spent on housing rose
rapidly. With respect to food, although proportionately less
was spent, people tended to consume more than they required
to meet their nutritional needs, although large households
with several children and pensioners were more likely to
obtain insufficient vitamins and protein because of low
incomes. Changing food consumption patterns could generated,
therefore, two different types of health problem: one
connected with potential obesity and the overconsumption of
animal fats and sugar, the other with possible malnutrition.
With respect to housing, the rapid rise in expenditure is in
part connected with the move to owner-occupation. In 1951 29
per cent of the housing built was in such occupation. This
figure had increased to 61 per cent by 1984.(4) Between 1961
and 1986, the numbers of households in owner occupation rose
from 7 millions to 14 millions.(5)

There have also been great improvements in housing amenities. In 1951 38 per cent of households in Britain were without the use of a fixed bath. The clearance and redevelopment schemes of local authorities, which it is now popular to malign, did much to improve this situation. The schemes provided purpose-built self-contained dwellings with all basic amenities on the basis of need. This - along with the activities of private house builders - meant that Britain is one of the best housed nations in Europe. Housing improvement has meant a great reduction in those lacking basic amenities like a fixed bath, inside toilet and so on. Their number fell from 2.8 m in 1971 to 0.9 m in 1981.(6) They fell even further between 1971 and 1985, from 12 to 2 per cent of all dwellings.(7) But the number of dwellings requiring repair, improvement or clearance has remained virtually the same for twenty years. In 1981, the figure stood at 2.1 m. In 1963 it was 2.5 m.(8) This does not mean that nothing has been done: simply that standards change so that higher ones must be met and that as some dwellings are improved, others fall behind. Today 'unfitness' is increasing in the owner-occupied sector, particularly as elderly owners cannot afford often essential repairs. This is disturbing for health, because of the strong association between quality of housing and state of health. Indeed this was recognised by the 1945 Labour government which placed housing under the remit of the Ministry of Health. This state of affairs lasted only until 1951. But in general we would assert that the housing improvements of the post-1945 period have made an important contribution to health second only to the sanitary reforms of the last half of the nineteenth century.

Important as it is for physical health, the home is also vital for mental health. The home is increasingly seen as a refuge, a haven where escape from the competitive, even destructive, forces of the wider world may be obtained. Britons are spending large proportions of their increasing leisure time in the home. In fact, Britain has the shortest hours worked of the EEC countries. There has also been an increase in the time people spend watching television - a 25 per cent rise between 1967 and 1979. In 1987, the average Briton watched just over 28 hours of television per week in the winter months. Video recorders are contributing to this leisure time - their ownership has increased rapidly, from one in five households in 1983 to one in three by 1985.(9) Other leisure pursuits are also family-centred, a trend no doubt assisted by the rise in car ownership. In 1947 33 per cent of households had use of a car. In 1985,the percentage had risen to 59, and in 1986 to 66.

What picture of Britain has emerged? Britain, in this overview, comes over as a prosperous society in which there is a narrowing of divisions. A gallup opinion poll conducted in 1977 discovered that by their own valuation, the British people were among the happiest in the world, while a New Society poll of the same year found that most were content with their economic lots - a finding common to all social classes - and were more concerned with the living of a

pleasant life than with working hard to accumulate more.(10)
Was Britain of the mid-1970s the new Jerusalem then? Was it
a place that truly represented a prosperous (in historic
rather than comparative terms) society of converging
individuals, who were all fast acquiring middle class
attitudes and attributes and who lived in a national that
could proclaim 'the end of ideology?'(11)

Of course, it was not. The apparent consensus of much of
the first 30 years of the post-1945 period could be said to
derive from an amalgam of ruling class complacency and working
class acceptance. The complacency emanates from the continued
domination of British society by a consolidated, coherent
upper class which enjoys disproportionate wealth, power and
life-chances.(12) The acceptance may be seen from the
increasing prosperity that we have just described. It does
not mean that working people accept all that is done to them
but what they have tended to accept is the means by which
prosperity is maintained and enhanced. Perceptive insights
on this process may be found in the work of Jeremy
Seabrook,(13) who has attempted to portray the nature and
effects of labour accepting the means (wage labour) and ends
(money) of capitalism. The post-war years have certainly seen
increases in wages and reductions in the burden of work, but
this bounty has led to the neglect of a deeper subordination
to the values of capitalism. The post-war years have
certainly seen increases in wages and reductions in the burden
of work, but his bounty has led to the neglect of a deeper
subordination to the values of capitalism. This attachment
of many workers to consumption(14) and to consumer capitalism
has remoulded everyday life. The market came to be
experienced as a provider with a greater emphasis on the
values of possessive individualism and privatism.(15)
Capitalism has 'captured' its working class not by coercion
but by, insidiously, unconsciously, providentially,
establishing that class's acceptance of its way of doing
things. Its way is not using coercive but ideological or
hegemonic.(16) By establishing its values as almost universal
in times of prosperity, it meant that the crises and
dislocations of the 1980s were met with acquiescence or
emulation. By pursuing economic betterment, therefore,
workers ignored the old solidarities that had got them through
hard times before. When the economic bubble burst, most were
ill-prepared for the difficulties that followed. Many of the
gains of the last thirty years would disappear exceedingly
quickly but the hegemony remains.

Poverty and ill-health did of course exist in Britain before
the mid-1970s. Indeed, they were 'rediscovered' in the
1960s.(17) But, for most and especially for policy-makers,
they were residual problems - ones that would disappear with
sufficient economic growth or by well-targeted welfare
benefits. We should not decry the optimism contained in such
sentiments. With economic growth and a benign, paternalistic,
directive state, everything seemed possible. But in the mid-
1970s the juggling act of trying to keep the balls of price
stability, full employment, high private sector profitability,

and stable balance of payments in the air failed.(18) High
public expenditure seen as necessary to maintain employment
opportunities and social welfare was increasingly the villain
of the piece squeezing out private investment, which would
bring 'real' jobs and 'real' prosperity. The post-1945
consensus on the mixed economy and the welfare state (19) was
destroyed, although the governing elements in both the Labour
and Conservative parties accepted the need for them to
maintain or create the conditions under which profitable
private accumulation was possible. And of course if more of
the surplus goes to profits less remains for wages and
salaries. Such a condition was found in circumstances where
more people were ready to compete on an individualist basis
for who should get what. In such circumstances, whatever the
level of prosperity, inequalities are likely to be enhanced,
especially when there is a government wedded to the notions
of individual enterprise and reward. The divisions in British
society became apparent again and widened further.

In saying that divisions became apparent again, we are
referring to and dealing with the dominant reality in British
society. It is a reality which has led to a growing pessimism
amongst Britons with respect to their standard and style of
living.(20) Many see a deterioration in elements of life that
touch them personally, such as riots, political terrorism and
safety on the streets. There is also a pessimism about the
likely benefit of economic policy although those in work are
fairly confident about their own job security and real
incomes, whereas the unemployed are sceptical about their own
job chances. Individually the relatively wealthy feel that
they have become wealthier, while the relatively poor see
themselves as poorer than before. In particular, local
authority tenants regard themselves (and are regarded by
others) as living in poor conditions and in a deteriorating,
iatrogenetic environment. These perceptions are accurate, or
more correctly, are borne out by changes in objective
conditions. Between 1976 and 1986 the distributions of income
and wealth have become more unequal. With respect to wealth,
state aid, particularly in the form of pensions, has had
little impact. The wealthiest half of the population
possesses 96 per cent of total wealth in 1983 (95 per cent in
1977). Between 1976 and 1985, the income share of the bottom
40.9 per cent fell from 10.2 to 6.3, while that of the top 20
per cent increased from 44.4 to 49.2. The gap is widening
rapidly. Between 1971 and 1986, a married couple with 2
children in the lowest 10 per cent of earners saw an average
increase of 18 per cent in their real disposable income. A
comparable family in the highest 10 per cent of earners saw
an average increase of some 31 per cent. With the linking of
pensions to prices rather than wages,the elderly have also
become worse off. At the same time, the housing budget has
been slashed by 70 per cent in real terms between 1979 and
1985,(21) meaning that few local authority dwellings are
constructed or repaired.

The opinion surveys note a differentiation in perceptions
between those in work and those unemployed. This is not

surprising. They miss the truncation of life chances brought about by the massive growth in unemployment. From 3.3 per cent in 1971 and 6.8 per cent in 1980, the unemployment figure rose to over 13.5 per cent by 1986. By the end of 1988, the official unemployment rate had fallen to 7.7 per cent, but this dramatic fall represents only a slight underlying decrease, the majority of the reduction being attributable to changes in the ways that unemployment is measured. By 1988, for example, no 16 to 18 year olds are included as they are considered to be in education or training if they have no work. These national figures also mark significant differences and divisions. The young and the older middle-aged are proportionately more likely to be unemployed. So too are black workers with those of West Indian descent being 2 1/2 times and those of Asian descent 1 1/2 times more likely to be unemployed than whites. There are large regional differences too with unemployment rates being 15.9 per cent in Northern Ireland, 10.2 in the North and 4.9 per cent in the South-east in 1988.

Unemployment is more likely to affect manual as opposed to non-manual workers. Between 1979 and 1984 2 1/2 m jobs were lost in manufacturing. Indeed in this period growth in services even stopped, although they had grown by some 2 m jobs between 1971 and 1979. In comparison over the entire period, jobs in the financial sector increased by some 40 per cent. Redundancies were also most felt in manufacturing. In 1982, the overall rate was 19.3 per 1000 employees. In manufacturing, it was 49.8 per 1000.

Other divisions may also be noted. The move towards more equal pay for men and women has been reversed. In 1983, women made up 40 per cent of workforce and 75 per cent of the low-paid.(22) Their earnings constituted only 75 per cent of those of men. By 1986, a full time female manual worker still earned only 62 per cent of the wage of a comparable male worker.(23)

Expenditure and consumption patterns also reveal important differences. 59 per cent of all households have the use of a car. But for those in work the figure is 76 per cent and for the self-employed 93 per cent. These compare with 37 per cent of the retired and 42 per cent of the unemployed.(24) While most social groups possessed a television and refrigerator, other household effects had a more differentiated pattern. 89 per cent of those in professional occupations compared with 68 per cent of unskilled workers possessed a washing machine in 1983. For a telephone and central heating, the respective figures are 95 and 53 per cent and 83 and 49 per cent. Those in the professional and management groups are also much more likely to own a video - 42 per cent compared with 18 per cent of manual workers.

We must remember that these divisions that we highlight are not independent ones. The divisions of class and employment, age, gender, race and region intersect to form coincidences of advantage or disadvantage with concomitant health problems.

"Britain is a divided society: a country partitioned by class, sex and race; a country of the employed and unemployed; a country of extraordinary personal wealth as well as continuing and widespread poverty".(25) For those in work, living standards continue to rise while the gradual dismemberment of the welfare services has adversely affected the poor, the unemployed and the sick. Britain is divided geographically with a prosperous south and less prosperous north, with the latter having fewer,more manual and more hazardous jobs. In the last ten years, the racial divisions in British society have worsened.(26) In the same period, the class divisions have become more stark: "right from the beginning of life, one's life chances,the chance of surviving birth, of suffering certain illnesses, the chances of living in certain types of accommodation, of receiving certain types of education and indeed the likelihood of earning a given income, are.. related to.. social classes. In fact, there seems to be very little life in our society which is not in some way characteristised by differences between social classes".(27)

Class, race, age, gender and locality form, therefore, significant dimensions of society. They are principles of social structure which shape social life.(28) Our own study is shaped by these principles and hence we have felt it important to characterise briefly how individuals with particular social attributes fare in Britain. On average, life is better for white, middle-aged men in professional jobs in the South-East than for any other type. But these structural dimensions do not have lives of their own. They define objectively a person's characteristics and social position. But we also give them meaning. We actively use the dimensions to shape our beliefs and perceptions on which we then act. There is, however, no easy two-way reciprocal relationship between structure and beliefs and perceptions. If we believe something to be true and/or right (even if it is not), that belief will affect the ways in which we behave. The exploration of the Western hemisphere was delayed because of the belief in a flat earth. So too if we believe that, say, class and race affect individual opportunity, then those beliefs will reinforce the objective determinations of class and race. In present-day britain, this reinforcement may be seen in the demoralisation and pessimism of much of the population. 70 per cent believe that class affects opportunity while 90 per cent believe that there is racial discrimination. Further, three-quarters feel that racial prejudice will increase or stay at its present level during the rest of the 1980s, and two-thirds are pessimistic about class divisions in the future.(29)

"Britain is a divided, demoralised, broken nation. Ours has become a nation in which the jobless are pitted against the employed; where the poor get poorer, while the rich get richer; where the wealthier South prospers at the expense of the impoverished North; where the sick suffer to benefit the healthy".(30) It is a sad but inevitable picture given the re-emergence of a rampant capitalism aided by a government that places the survival and growth of the system above the needs of individuals. The social divisions based on class, age, gender, race and locality that lay submerged beneath (or were seen as treatable by) the mixed economy-welfare state consensus have also gained renewed prominence. They are divisions that greatly shape all life chances, e.g. employment, housing, education and health. We shall turn, therefore, to how these divisions are played out in the health sector.

INEQUALITIES IN HEALTH

"There is so much evidence demonstrating differences in mortality and morbidity between the social classes.. that it is difficult to select from the evidence".(31) The Department of Health and Social Security Report - the Black Report - documented these differences.(32) It discovered that class differences in mortality are a constant feature of the entire human lifetime though these differences are more marked at the start of life and in early adulthood. At birth and during the first month of life the risk of death in the unskilled manual group is double the risk in the professional group. The greatest differences are found in deaths resulting from accidents and respiratory disease, causes of death which are associated with the social economic-environment. Class disadvantage does become less extreme with increasing age and with adulthood, causes of death become extremely varied and there are significant gender differences in addition to those of class. Thus circulatory disease, nutritional and metabolic diseases of the digestive system affect working class women most severely and malignant neoplasms, accidents and diseases of the nervous system working class men. Diseases in which class is significant for both sexes include the infective and parasitic, those of the blood and blood-forming organs, those of the genito-urinary systems and, most important, diseases of the respiratory system.

Although mortality rates have declined over the last 100 years, there is little evidence to suggest that social class differences in mortality are at present lessening. In fact, the position of unskilled manual workers is deteriorating in relation to certain diseases. The 'old' diseases - those of poverty (e.g. bronchitis, respiratory tuberculosis) - show a widening gap between the classes while the diseases of affluence - diabetes, coronary disease - are also increasingly concentrated in the lowest two classes, as is lung cancer. This may well point to the different impact of health education among the classes. Death rates from some causes are higher in the higher classes - leukaemia, cancer of the breast, cirrhosis of the liver. Overall, the annual risk of death for men is considerably higher in the lower social classes. In 1986, the SMR for professional workers was 63; for the unskilled it was 131.(33) And the social class differences have continued to widen almost continuously since 1951.(34)

It is more difficult to chart the quantity and distribution of sickness and ill-health. But class differences are more likely to occur in chronic rather than acute illnesses, with prevalence rates being three times as great in Class V as in Class I. The average number of days lost from work through illness or accident is more than four times higher among unskilled manual male workers than among professional men. In fact, incapacity for work rates increase for all conditions from social Class I to V, the respective rates being, for example, 91 per 1000 to 177 per 1000 for diseases of the respiratory system, 7 to 40 per 1000 for arthritis and 15 to 57 per 1000 for bronchitis. There has though been a general and progressive increase in the number of people reporting chronic (long-standing) sickness from 1972 to 1986. There is variation between socio-economic groups. Thus 23 per cent of men and 21 per cent of women in professional occupations reported chronic sickness compared with 35 per cent of men and 42 per cent of women in unskilled manual occupations. There is though a decline in the relative differences as prevalence is increasing more rapidly in the professional group.(36) Rates of restricted activity are less clearly differentiated along class lines. Specific illnesses are so differentiated e.g. childhood infectious diseases and dental health. There also appear to be class variations in psychiatric disorders, although the relationship is not straightforward and there are problems with the data and the definitions of what constitutes mental disorder.(37)

Inequalities in health status by other social dimensions are less easily discerned than those by class because of the lack of available data and the interrelationships between the dimensions. Standardised mortality rates (standardised for age and class) have been worked out for the regions of England and Wales. They show that in terms of mortality, the healthiest part of Britain appears to be the belt south of a line drawn from the Wash to the Bristol Channel.(38) The relationship between health and ethnicity has not been firmly established. Much work has, in the past, concentrated on the 'special' needs of ethnic minorities in terms of sickle cell anaemia and thalassaemia.(39) The notion that black people can be assumed to have higher than average rates of mortality and morbidity because of general economic and social disadvantage is difficult to test. Many of the associations are inferred from data on class-related inequalities and further research is required.(40)

There also exist inequalities in access to and use of health care facilities. No significant ethnic disadvantage has been noted for the use of general practitioners and ante-natal clinics at least.(41) Significant class inequalities do, however, emerge. The Black Report showed that there are higher consultation rates for manual workers (for both men and women) than non-manual workers when all age groups are considered. This does not, however, mean that manual workers are using GPs at the rate which the mortality and morbidity data suggest they should. Attempts have been made to develop use-to-need ratios. These establish that manual workers use

GP services less in relation to needs than non-manual workers. The meaning and interpretation of consultation rates are still the subject of debate.(42) In the case of hospital services there is little evidence with which to evaluate the effect of social class on utilisation. Some Scottish data suggest that hospital admission rates and length of hospital stay increased from social class I to V.(43) Unskilled males also tend to use outpatient departments more than other males. This may be related to occupational hazard being greater for these men than others. The strongest evidence of the underutilisation of services by manual workers and their families can be found in the preventive and promotional services e.g. antenatal clinic attendance, dental visits, immunisation. It appears too that health education and promotion (because of the nature of its approach) is less effective among such people if the differential rates for smoking and obesity are relevant measures. The number of adult smokers is now down to one in three, but this hides considerable class differences: 17 per cent of professional men smoke compared with 49 per cent of unskilled men.

There are also geographical variations in access to health care facilities. Studies in the mid-1970s pointed to the strong association between the percentage of the population in professional and managerial occupations and high levels of regional expenditure on hospital and community health services.(44) Thus the social class composition of a region affected the quantity and quality of services. As resources are all located on a regional basis, these findings form the basis of attempts to redistribute funds and facilities in favour of the poorer regions, and hence the lower social classes. From the mid-1970s on, health inequalities became the subject of health care policy as well as academic debate.

POLICIES FOR RESOURCE ALLOCATION AND HEALTH EDUCATION

For our purposes, we can say that health care policy for resource redistribution took two forms. The first was to attempt to move resources from acute services towards the so-called 'Cinderella Services', those caring for the elderly, the mentally infirm and the mentally handicapped. The aim though was to devolve away from the hospital to the community in order to provide a more therapeutic setting for treatment.(45) The second, referred to at the end of the last section, concerned regional reallocation. The DHSS set up a working party - the Resource Allocation Working Party (RAWP) - to establish criteria for creating equal opportunity of access to health care for people at equal risk. The criteria were meant to be responsive to relative need, rather than supply or demand. While there are some problems in this approach, e.g. health care was equated with hospital care for the most part and need was measured by standardised mortality rates rather than morbidity, RAWP was meant to achieve a redistribution in favour of the relatively deprived regions, primarily those in the North. The priority of the Cinderella Services could be worked out within the RAWP formulations at the regional level. As initially formulated, there were to be no 'losers' in these attempts at redistribution. The relatively deprived would be positively discriminated against in that they would receive more than their 'fair share' of growth money. It did not quite turn out like that. The RAWP and priority programme formulations coincided with the economic crisis outlined above and with the arrival of a Conservative Government dedicated to rolling back the state.

RAWP developed as a technical device to allocate financial resources. Such a device can be used to redistribute additional funds or to decide where to cut from static or declining budgets. Up to 1983-4, there had been some redistribution in favour of the relatively deprived regions.(46) But these 'gains' had been obtained at the expense of real cuts in health care provision particularly in the London health regions.(47) In 1986-8, the policy was thoroughly reviewed.(48) Principal recommendations include improving the use of mortality statistics and the incorporation of a measure of social deprivation to make the formula more sensitive to health needs. These suggested changes have proved somewhat controversial and are being debated, but so far have slowed the pace of cuts in the London health regions because these tend to score highly in terms of overall social deprivation.

The policy of cost containment and reduction may also be seen in the deinstitutionalisation of care for the elderly and the mentally infirm and handicapped. Deinstitutionalisation allows for the saving of resources as well as their transfer from the hospital sector to community services. Community care has fast become family care. Further, health education has become a matter of exhortation with the Health Education Council's largest campaign in 1984 against smoking receiving under 3/4 million pounds.(49) While it is debatable whether exhortation is more likely to reduce the level of smoking as opposed to increases in excise duty, this is a paltry sum given the resistance to change among certain groups of smokers. For them smoking is beneficial and this may allow them to define away the medical opinions on the deleterious effects of smoking as our own study shows.

Cost containment has meant a disintegrating, shabbier health service in most places and for most people. In real terms, allowing for inflation, demographic change (our ageing population) and technological developments, the health authority budgets were cut by 2 per cent or so between 1979 and 1984.(50) The only real growth has been in family practitioner services which have not as yet been cash-limited as these services are demand-generated and not supply-determined. It is possible (to reduce hospital beds (and lengthen waiting lists and/or reduce length of stay) but not possible to limit the number of visits a person makes to her/his GP's surgery. These calculations, however, give the lie of claims on above-inflation expenditure on the NHS. It is not so much a case of doing better and feeling worse but doing worse and feeling it. This must be in part responsible for the fact that just under half of those questioned for the

British social attitudes report thought that the NHS was well run.(51) This compares with 85 per cent who thought the banks were well run, 72 per cent the police, 33 per cent local government and 20 per cent nationalised industries. By 1988, however, only 6 per cent were completely happy with the way the NHS was being run as controversy over government plans took centre stage. Specific complaints about NHS services are rising, being highest of all amongst the higher social classes.(52) But the changing attitudes we noted above with the psychic subordination of the working class to capitalism, may be seen in health care. While 30 per cent thought that private medicine was a good thing for the NHS, 68 per cent rejected the idea that the NHS should be available free only to the poorest section of the population with the rest being covered by private health schemes. By 1986, one in 10 households were covered by private medical insurance, although there are great variations between social classes and regions.

CONCLUSIONS

There is then an association between objective conditions and people's actions and perceptions. We cannot just assume that because a particular state of affairs exists then individuals will automatically think and act in a particular way. The brief appraisals of life in Britain and health inequalities are the frameworks within which people's lives (including their health statuses and uses of health care facilities) take place. We have seen how these frameworks have led to various policy formulations, the goals of which have changed over the last ten years from the pursuit of equity to cost containment. Again these policies form a backdrop against which people assess their health and use facilities. But use is not only dependent on the supply of resources. It is also shaped by people's own assessments of their health and their needs. While life in Britain will affect these assessments as we show in Chapter 4, these assessments affect consultation and utilisation rates and through these, feeding as they do into policy, resource allocation. People's perceptions of their health are also likely to affect their responses to health education programmes such as those directed towards healthy eating and against smoking. What people think of their health and what causes and cures illness are, therefore, vital elements in the process of seeking help and should so be seen in the formulation of policy. We shall return briefly to policy in the final chapter but shall now concentrate on health perceptions and attitudes to care. Our study looks at working class and black health because these are the groups which suffer most in terms of health inequalities and how life in Britain is presently constituted. Further, we examine the health perceptions of individuals with these social attributes in different regional contexts - the North (West Yorkshire), the Midlands (Greater Birmingham) and the South (London). We shall explain our choice of study areas in the next chapter. We selected different areas because we did not know if there were likely to be any differences in perceptions. But the importance of these perceptions and beliefs cannot be dismissed. A sense of well-being is crucial to good health and vital for policy if individuals are to be persuaded to become more responsible for their own well-being.(53) It seemed (and still seems) worthwhile trying to find out if differences in perceptions exist. We do not pretend, however, that we are the first to look at health and health care perceptions. These other studies will open Chapter 2.

FOOTNOTES

1. Many studies employing subjective social indicators (that is measures which try to establish what people think of aspects of life) show that health is often ranked first in order of importance above standard of living, job, family life and so on. Many of these studies are reported in the journal <u>Social Indicators Research</u>.

2. The account which follows derives largely from S. Toland, changes in living standards since the 1950s, <u>Social Trends</u> 10, 1980, 13-38 and A Marwick, <u>British Society Since 1945</u>, Penguin, 1982.

3. The extension of benefits to a wide range of disabled and disadvantaged groups in the 1960s and early 1970s is described by P. Townsend, <u>Poverty in the United Kingdom</u>, Penguin, 1979, chapters 24 to 27.

4. Figures derived form <u>Social Trends</u> 16, 1986.

5. Figures from <u>Social Trends</u>, 18, 1988.

6. Department of the Environment, <u>English housing condition survey 1981</u>, DOE, 1984.

7. Figures form <u>Social Trends</u>, 18, 1988.

8. J. Eyles, Area-based policies for the inner city in D. Herbert and D. M. smith (eds.) <u>Social problems and the city</u>, Oxford UP, 1979.

9. Figures form <u>Social Trends</u>, 18, 1988.

10. These surveys of opinion are quoted in Marwick <u>op.cit</u>.

11. Throughout the 1950s and 1960s much was made of the possible social consequences of increased working class wages. It was thought then the working class would begin to take on not only middle class life-styles but also attitudes. This 'embourgeoisement' of the working class would result in a one-class society - 'we are all middle class now' - where ideological differences would disappear. It would indeed be the end of ideology. Much of this debate, its problems and bases for its ultimate rejection are provided in J. Goldthorpe et al., <u>The affluent worker in the class structure</u>, Cambridge UP, 1969. Reality - among the car workers Goldthorpe and his colleagues studied - demonstrated that the idea of a developing 'classlessness' was false.

12. On this domination, see Marwick <u>op cit</u>, A. Marwick, <u>Class,image and reality</u>, Fontana, 1980; J. Westergard and H. Resler, <u>Class in a capitalist society</u>, Penguin, 1975.

13. J. Seabrook, <u>Unemployment</u>, Paladin, 1982.

14. On this shift to consumerism see J. Alt, Beyond class, _Telos_ 28, 1976, 55-80.

15. These values are highlighted too by S. Hall, The culture gap, _Marxism Today_ 28(1), 1984, 18-22.

16. Hegemony is a notion deriving from the Italian marxist Antonio Gramsci and represents the domination of society through ideas, values, ways of seeing and doing rather than just coercion. For commentaries see C. Boggs, _Gramsci's marxism_, Pluto Press 1976; R. Simon, _Gramsci's political thought_, Lawrence and Wishart, 1982.

17. Interesting studies that helped this rediscovery includes E. Coates and R. Silburn, _Poverty: the forgotten Englishmen_, Penguin, 1970; Townsend _op cit_, B. Abel-Smith and P. Townsend, _The poor and the poorest_, Bell, 1965.

18. This combination of problems is well analysed by A Gamble and P. Walton, _Capitalism and crisis_, Macmillan, 1976.

19. The break-up of the post-war consensus with respect to welfare is discussed by R. Mishra, _The welfare state in crisis_, Wheatsheaf, 1984.

20. These attitudes are charted in R. Jowell and C. Airey (eds.) _British social attitudes: the 1984 report_, Gower, 1985; and R. Jowell, C. Witherspoon and P. Brook (eds.) _British Social Attitudes: The Fifth Report_, Gower, 1988.

21. H.M. Treasury, _Government expenditure plans_, HMSO, 1986.

22. Figures from T. Manwaring and N. Sigler (eds) _Breaking the nation_, Pluto Press, 1985.

23. Figures from _Social Trends_, 18, 1988.

24. _Social Trends_ 15, 1985.

25. S. Fothergill and J. Vincent, _The state of the nation_, Pan. 1985, 7.

26. See C. Brown, _Black and white Britain_, Heinemann, 1984.

27. I. Reid, _Social class differences in Britain_,   Grant McIntyre, 1981, 298.

28. The idea that there are specific social dimensions that structure social life is well developed in social theory. In recent times attempts have been made to incorporate the notion that these 'structures' are not simply 'out there' but are created by human activity, which once they are created, they affect.   There is then a complex relationship between that which is created, how, and on what basis it is created and the structures themselves. This relationship has been summarised as the mutual dependence of agency and structure in the theory of

structuration. This theory was developed in the main by A. Giddens. <u>The constitution of society</u>, Polity Press, 1984 but is also paralleled in the work of R. Bhaskar, <u>The possibility of naturalism</u>, Harvester, 1979.

29. Jowell and Airey <u>op cit</u>.

30 Manwaring and Sigler <u>op cit</u>, 1.

31. J. Brotherson, Inequality: is it inevitable? in C.O. Carter and J. Peel (eds) <u>Equalities and inequalities in health</u>, Academic Press, 1976, 73.

32. Department of Health and Social Security, <u>Inequalities in health</u>, DHSS, 1980. Only 260 duplicated copies of the typescript were made publicly available in the week of the August Bank Holiday. A slimmed-down version was produced was produced by P. Townsend and N. Davidson, <u>Inequalities in health</u>, Penguin, 1982. On inequalities see also L. Doyal, <u>The political economy of health</u>, Pluto Press, 1979; V. Walters, <u>Class inequality and health care</u>, Croom Helm, 1980; J. Eyles and K.J. Woods, <u>The social geography of medicine and health</u>, Croom Helm, 1983.

33. Figures from <u>Social Trends</u>, 18, 1988.

34. See M.A. Marmot, Mortality decline and widening social inequalities, <u>Lancet</u> ii, 1986, 276-6. Health Education Council, <u>The health divide</u>, HEC 1987; A Smith and B. Jacobson (eds.) <u>The nation's health</u>, Kings Fund, 1988.

35. Reid <u>op cit</u>.

36. <u>Social Trends</u> 14, 1984.

37. See, for example, M. Rutter and N. Madge, <u>Cycles of disadvantage</u>, Heinemann, 1976, and R. Littlewood and M. Lipsedge, <u>Aliens and alienists</u>, Penguin, 1982.

38. Townsend and Davidson <u>op cit</u>. <u>Social Trends</u> 18, 1988, Smith and Jacobson <u>op cit</u>.

39. J. Donovan, Ethnicity and health: a research review, <u>Social Science and Medicine</u> 19, 1984, 663-70; R. Fitzpatrick, <u>The experience of illness</u>, Tavistock, 1984; T. Rathwell and D. Phillips (eds.) <u>Health, race and ethnicity</u>, Croom Helm 1986.

40. See Townsend and Davidson <u>op cit</u>.

41. Brown <u>op cit</u>. But in a more recent study of GP consultation, it was found that patients of Afro-Caribbean descent received less detailed explanations than others from their doctors. See D.A. Tuckett et al., <u>Meetings between experts</u>, Tavistock, 1986.

42. E. Collins and R. Klein, Equity and the NHS, British Medical Journal 281, 1980, 1111-5.

43. V. Carstairs and P.E. Patterson, Distribution of hospital patients by social class, Health Bulletin 24, 1966, 59-65.

44. J. Noyce et al., Regional variations in the allocation of financial resources to the community health services, Lancet 1, 1975, 345-7; J.E. Rickard, Per capita expenditure of English area health authorities, British Medical Journal 277, 1976, 299-300.

45. See, for example, P. Abrams, Community care, Policy and Politics 6, 1977. 125-51; J. Allsop, Health policy and the NHS, Longman, 1984, J.R. Butler and M. Vaile, Health and health services, RKP, 1984.

46. See Office of Health Economics, Compendium of health statistics (5th Edition), OHE. 1984.

47. See J. Mohan and K.J. Woods, Restructuring health care, International Journal of Health services 15, 1985, 197-215.

48. For details see DHSS Review of RAWP Formula, 1988.

49. J. Eyles and K.J. Woods, Who cares what care, Social Science and Medicine 23, 1986, 1087-92.

50. See Manwaring and Sigler op cit.

51. Jowell and Airey op cit.

52. See Jowell et al. (eds.) British Social Attitudes: The Fifth Report, Gower, 1988.

53. Self-help and individual responsibility are important components of most health promotion strategies in the 1980s. See J. Eyles The geography of the national health, Croom Helm, 1987 for a summary and Smith and Jacobson op cit.

2 Perceptions of health and illness

In carrying out our research in what white working class and black people think about their health and health care, we work within what is known as 'the interpretative paradigm' which "manages to acknowledge the existence of medical power without turning patients into passive, acquiescent or dependent victims. Patients, all social actors, are seen as people who actively and creatively produce and reproduce the meanings that sustain their social world in every moment of their interactions with other people".(1) This may not sound particularly unusual. Commonsense tells us that we help create and maintain our social relationships and institutions by our own thoughts and actions. It is quite unusual, however, for much social science research on health and illness. This research sees our everyday, commonplace perceptions as unscientific or ideologically suspect.(2) Interpretative research allows our perceptions and concepts to be treated as important, meaningful phenomena in their own right, influencing behaviour and shaping the social world. It does also mean, however, that the contexts of these perceptions and concepts are extremely important. It is false to try to pretend that such beliefs exist in a vacuum. They are part and parcel of everyday material reality. By taking on board the context of beliefs, we are able to see that certain beliefs and actions are rational in terms of context. So when some people of Afro-Caribbean descent reject pills as medication and express a strong preference for liquids, their view is not unscientific but perfectly rational in the context of their culture and the theories of bodily operation on which they are based. Further, smoking is not irrational among certain sections of the white working class, but it provides a way of coping, of relieving the stresses and strains of work and home life. That makes smoking in such a context a supremely rational act.

The interpretative approach leads, therefore, to the serious examination of perceptions of health, health care and illness. If we are interested in the meanings people use to understand situations and how social context will affect the quality of their lives, proper analysis can also be undertaken of lay explanations of illness and how their views of life in Britain affect them. But while the interpretative approach has a long history in social philosophy,(3) it has not as yet generated much empirical research. There have been studies of disability and handicap(4) and of patients in medical settings,(5) but those of individuals in the general population are of recent origin. There is a fairly widespread agreement that lay beliefs are complex and consist of many different factors.(6) There are though common themes - perhaps the least surprising of which is that people's conceptions of health and illness are medical. They are after all, regardless of class background and country of origin, part of a shared medicalised, industrial culture.(7) This is not, however, to say that lay and medical beliefs coincide. Lay people have great difficulty in defining health, except in terms of an absence of disease or illness. The facts that the experiences and references of lay person and professional are separate are grounds for conflicts of perspectives.(8) But the gulf between the 'two sides' should not be overstated. Of course, religion may be seen as a cause or relief of particular illnesses as the women of Afro-Caribbean descent in our own study demonstrate, but the medicalisation of everyday life(9) means that lay people are conversant with many medical terms. Further, doctors do not always apply the models of particular complaint description and causation presented in text books. It has been found, for example, that practising gynaecologists' views of the menopause were based on few and selective scientific principles. There was also a wide variety of approaches from the biomedical to the psychosocial.(10) Doctors are also people, and they may retain many lay assumptions about illness and disease.(11) But the possibility of confusion and conflict between medical and lay beliefs remains with the same term not necessarily meaning the same thing to both parties.(12)

In our own work, however, we are not so much concerned with those differences as with lay beliefs themselves in the sense that a belief truly held will have consequences for individual actions. We are also concerned with putting these beliefs into the social contexts from which they derive, because contexts will shape the nature and effect of beliefs. In this, our work shares some of the same aims of that of Cornwell(13) and Roberts.(14) Cornwell in her study of health and illness in Bethnal Green quite rightly suggests that it is not enough to know that health is interpreted as functional ability or capacity for work without knowing about people's work. In Bethnal Green she found that men and women share a common view on work and its meaning but that there are significant differences between them that affect their reactions to ill-health. For men, 'work' means paid employment, while for the women, many of whom are also in such employment, work means housework and childcare. Men worked as long as they were able to but if they stayed away from work they expected the women to look after them often to a chorus of complaints from the women. Women did not try to work off symptoms as men often did but tried to contain the symptoms to keep going. They slowed down and cut out certain activities rather than giving up altogether. Similar attitudes are found by Roberts in her study of women and their doctors. They must not only look after the home and children as 'housewives' but they are the ones who care and nurture, being responsible for health within the family.

Many of the studies we have cited point also to the variety and significance of lay ideas about the causes of illnesses. Infection or germs tended to be the most commonly cited cause.(15) Also important, particularly in studies of women in both Scotland and South Wales, were life-style and heredity. Environmental hazards, individual responsibility and stress were further causes. The last named, stress, is seen as a characteristic way of interpreting ill-health and 'worry' figures prominently in our own account in Chapter 3. We should note, however, that there is no universal agreement as to that which causes illness. Further, the same environment may be seen as illness-producing or health-enhancing or merely neutral by different individuals. So the context of everyday life which is very often seen as the 'cause' of sickness is not static, unitary or universal. People's perceptions of it vary, depending on their own individual attributes, circumstances and culture. In this way, lay beliefs are derived which treat the same phenomena in different ways. So, for example, while virtually all individuals see diet as a contributory factor for health and illness, it is viewed variably. This may be seen most clearly if cross-cultural comparisons are made. There remain people of Asian descent who regard a fat child as a healthy child and, therefore, western views on obesity and 'overeating' as wrong-headed. Within the white population, there are variations in what is considered to be sufficient exercise to remain healthy. In our study, many of those who performed what they considered to be a full load in paid employment or housework or childcare thought they did enough exercise in their jobs although they would not ensure the burning off of excessive calories.

Other work has made the distinction in causes of illness between behaviour, i.e. that which is the individual's own responsibility, and environment or circumstances, i.e. that which is outside the individual's immediate control.(16) We feel that this is a useful distinction and indeed employ it ourselves, although it is impossible to draw a hard and fast line between the two. They not only merge with one another but also interact with, and subtly alter, one another as well. Blaxter's research, however, found behaviour to be mentioned about four times more often than circumstances as causing ill health. Thus smoking, diet, exercise and mental state were more frequently cited than environmental factors. This should perhaps not surprise us. 'Behaviour' is more immediate, specific and personal to individuals that 'circumstances' which seem perhaps general, remote and simply 'there'. For this reason, we have chosen to isolate and discuss in full the broad context of people's lives and health as we did in Chapter 1. For our respondents, this context is examined in Chapter 4 in terms of the parameters of life in Britain that people see as affecting the way they live, their quality of life and their health. Work and racism have particular salience. So too does locality or neighbourhood, although this is discussed as part of environment in Chapter 3 because it is the immediate area, the home of potential germs and the place which, to some extent, may be shaped and controlled by the individual.

This distinction of behaviour and circumstances is related to another way of distinguishing 'causes', namely public and private theories.(17) 'Public' explanations usually include a reference to the medical profession as in 'they say' or 'I've heard'. This reference allows for the identification of the external agent or combination of internal and external mechanisms in causation. It also usually means that the illness is seen as unavoidable - or in terms of the previous discussion, beyond our immediate control - so the person with the disease cannot be blamed for having it. Such disease is regarded almost as a 'natural' outcome of life. This in itself may lead to a fatalistic or acquiescent reaction to certain types of illness, although as we shall see the types vary from individual to individual. 'Private' explanations, on the other hand, appeal only to the authority of the speaker or a close friend or relative. Such accounts are often hesitant and take the form of story-telling in which life history or life style are prominent. Private theories emphasise a causal process in which there is movement between factors internal to a person and those outside them and in their environment. The causes of illness are thus known about rather than known. Fluid, individual circumstances are at the centre of private theories. This leads Cornwell to conclude that no statements can be made about the avoidability of, and responsibility and blame for, an illness. We disagree. As Chapter 3 shows, depending on individual circumstances, people can make their own luck with respect to illness and disease; they are seen as being able to determine in some measure, their own life-styles. Some then appear to be blamed for going down with unavoidable illnesses. If it is their fault then treatment may not be compassionate. This view is also increasingly held by policy-makers in medicine and government, who regard 'unhealthy' behaviours as avoidable and easily changed. In Britain part of the strategy for the 1990s is to promote 'lifestyles for health.'(18) The report recognises, however, the importance of public action. But, further, lay and expert opinion on healthy behaviour may vary. Thus because of these types of problem, and the merging of public and private theories, we do not find the distinction as useful as the one between 'behaviour' and 'circumstances' although Roberts in examining illness causation in women uses the distinction between 'old wives' tales' and 'old doctor's tales'(19), a variant, it would seem, on the private-public theme.

In these studies then we see many of the themes emerging
that will appear in the ensuing chapters - concepts of health
and illness, causes of ill health, context of health and
illness. We feel that our treatment is somewhat different
from the other individual studies in that we try to amalgamate
consideration of cause and context, seeing concepts as the
backdrop against which the other issues are considered. Like
several of the other studies, we also consider the health care
system. We are more concerned with the perceptions people
have of their doctors and hospitals(20) but recognise that
these perceptions are related to the experiences people have
as patients, visitors and general 'consumers' of health
care.(21) As we stated in Chapter 1, we consider these views
important for policy as well as academic reasons. But before
we come to the presentation of our material, we feel that we
must briefly state how it was obtained.

METHOD

We have already said that our research is located within the
'interpretative paradigm' - an emphasis on meanings and the
social construction of the world - and this imposes in itself
certain methodological constraints. There are, however, other
ways of obtaining data on what people think their health
status is and how they use the health services. It is
possible to use structured survey instruments. These consist
of an established set of questions which are asked in the same
order and ways of every individual. The questions may have
a limited number of responses and the individual has to check
the one that is closest to her/his own view. They may also
take the form of statements about health status or level of
satisfaction with the health services. If the questionnaire
takes the form of a series of statements, respondents are
usually required to say where they fall on a scale of opinion
from strongly agree to strongly disagree or mostly true to
mostly not true. Some statement series demand simpler
answers, such as a yes or no. So, for example, individuals
are asked to respond strongly agree - mostly agree - not sure
-mostly disagree - strongly disagree to such statements as
'doctors always treat their patients with respect' and 'It's
hard to get an appointment for health care straight-away'.(22)
They are asked to check one of definitely true - mostly true -
don't know - mostly false - definitely false to such items
as 'I'm not as healthy now as I used to be' and 'I've never
had an illness that lasted a long time.(23) A yes or no
response is required to such statements as 'I'm feeling on
edge', 'I'm tired all the time', and 'I'm finding it hard to
make contact with people'. If respondents are unsure, they
are asked to say which is more true at the moment.(24)

Such instruments have been through rigorous trials to ensure
that they are as meaningful as they can be to individual
respondents. If a checklist of answers is provided, the
answers suggested have to be mutually exclusive and represent
real choices in the everyday lives of those being interviewed.
While these instruments may impose meaning on social relations
through their prior definitions and lead to the need for ex

post facto interpretation of unexpected findings.(25) They seem useful for collecting factual information e.g. how often a particular service is used by individuals with different social attributes. The health section of the General Household Survey is an example of a structured survey instrument. It does also ask opinion questions but requires fairly straightforward answers of the type - good, not so good, don't know.(26)

Structured questionnaires are also used to elicit information on perceived health status, views on health, illness and illness causation and attitudes to health care provision. Their advantages are that they are fairly easy to administer (though not construct), may be utilised by a team of researchers as the question sequence and wording are fixed and can be directed at large numbers of people. This last-named attribute is extremely important because it mean that a representative sample of the population group(s), in which the researcher is interested, can be obtained. This in turn means that the findings can be presented as statistically significant generalisations, a practice which social science has borrowed from the natural sciences.

These benefits are bought at what we would regard as considerable cost. With the series of statements, the same end-product - the score which represents a person's health status or attitude to health care - may be achieved in very different ways.(27) Once given, the answer to a statement tends to become divorced from its context or any expressed doubts. In fact, an individual in responding to a statement is asked to suspend any doubts and provide a categorical answer which the researcher can then authoritatively interpret.(28) These doubts though arise with respect to context and meaning. It must be assumed in constructing the statements that once they are established they are context-independent. In other words, it does not matter what the specific circumstances of individuals are,they will all answer in a systematic way. Further, it assumed that the items means the same to all individuals. So the statements have to assume that individual circumstances and experiences can be encompassed by one-word answers and that words like 'satisfied', 'conveniently', 'seriously', 'painful' are crystal clear. Our experience is that this is not the case. One statement which can, for example, cause specific difficulties is 'I'm waking up in the early hours of the morning'. It is meant to discover sleep and energy problems. But shorn of its context, a worker on early shift or a parent with a child requiring medication could and did respond 'yes' without any personal health problems. We cite two further examples from our work:

Sheila (Parkheath); [doctors don't advise patients about ways to avoid illness and injury.] I dunno. What do I put there? I think he would tell you if it was your fault... Doctors aren't as thorough as they should be. I don't know what that means. My doctor is quick, but the hospitals aren't.

Doreen (Parkheath): [I have never been seriously ill.] Do you call heart trouble serious?... I suppose at the time it was. At that time - well, no, I wasn't <u>seriously</u> ill before, I just couldn't do things and I wasn't seriously ill after the operation. But at the time of the operation, I had a relapse and had to be dashed to the operating theatre. But that is only, to me, one instance... To me, I'm OK with the checkups at the hospital, if I take my time and don't do anything silly... to me, a serious illness is prolonged... Help me! I have never been seriously ill. Mostly true. It is difficult. Anybody that suffers with, like emphysema - that, to me, is terrible.

Such debate is usually lost with a structured instrument. Many of our respondents told such stories when they tried to answer the opinion statements. Of course, we recognise that it must be 'horses for courses': that any measure of health depends on the purpose for which it is required as well as the audience that makes us of it. We further note that there is no hard-and-fast line between different types of survey and that they can inform each other.(29) But we would argue that we still know very little about lay beliefs, this being shown in the different, if related, ways in which they are structured by social scientists. In this case then intensive interviews with a relatively small number of people may still be an extremely significant way forward.

Intensive interviews involve the researcher in talking to individuals on a wide variety of topics relevant to the matter at hand. The suitability of the topics is discovered beforehand in much the same way as a structured survey instrument is tested. But the end-product of this piloting is not definitive question wording and sequencing. Rather, it is a check list of topics to be covered with each respondent. They may be put to the individual in any order and in any form. The role of the interviewer is, therefore, crucial as are her/his attributes. She/he must be an empathetic listener and a good conversationalist - indeed Sidney and Beatrice Webb referred to interviewing as 'conversation with a purpose'.(30) The researcher must recognise the artificiality of most interview settings and, therefore, the likelihood that certain types of conversation will go unrecorded. This recognition may lead the researcher to adopt other strategies, participant observation for example, and that her/his data are limited.(31) Further, she/he needs also to be a knowledgeable social theorist so that information may be linked with concepts to try and develop understanding and explanation in more general terms.

Intensive interviews have variously been called field work, field research, interpretative social science, qualitative methods and ethnography. Their intensive nature and establishment lead to particular problems which further limit the numbers of people that can be 'interviewed'. There may be, for example, problems of access to particular individuals (how do you go about finding black respondents with the required social attributes?) and entry to specific settings (how does a male researcher enter a mothers-and-toddlers (sic) group?). If it is the intention of the research to discuss at length, say, health topics and those of related interest (which specify the context) then the conversations are likely to take a long time. Ours varied from thirty minutes to about three hours. It may also be necessary to go back to individuals to clarify points or take the discussions further. Two sets of interviews were in fact carried out with those of both Afro-Caribbean and Asian descent. It is usual to tape record all the conversations with all the individuals so everything spoken, including tone and inflection, is available for analysis at later dates. All that is taped has to be transcribed. A rough estimate of transcription time is that it takes five minutes to transcribe one minute of taped conversation. Our three white working class groups generated 85 hours of tape, meaning that transcription took something like 10 working weeks. There are then practical limits to how many individuals can be intensively interviewed. There are also substantive reasons why the numbers are and should be limited.

These reasons are perhaps best treated in a brief discussion about representativeness. A question frequently raised by those more familiar with natural science methods and statistical generalisation is what can you meaningfully say on the basis of 20 or 30 interviews? Cornwell's study involved 24 including the pilot stage, Donovan's of black health a total of 30 and our three regional 'surveys' only 110. The answer is that you can say a great deal, but it cannot, is not nor should be, couched in terms of representativeness. What is said takes the form of a descriptive and theoretical account of the presented material.(32) The aim is to obtain a very high level of detail so that a segment of the world is known thoroughly. It is further known in the terms (the meanings) of individual respondents. While in some respects these terms are unique to individuals in that at one level all our lives differ in some respects, common themes begin to emerge which form the basis of generalisation. After a while, talking with further individuals will cease to lead to the emergence of new themes. This is the point at which the limit to the number interviewed may be discerned substantively. The common themes are of course found in what people say, in their stories of their lives and those of others, but those stories are interpreted and structured by the researcher. Thus the aim of this approach is to produce theoretical and descriptive generalisations which emerge form a thorough investigation of part of the world. How such generalisations emerge in our interpretations must be briefly considered.

We recognise that many individuals create, maintain and change the meanings that the world has for them not necessarily directly (as in the commitment to the American way in every American school at morning prayers) but indirectly through telling stories. According to Heller,(33) telling stories is a way that people make sense of everyday life. The researcher essentially listens to these stories that people recount from and about their lives. The stories are concerned with what the world is like rather than abstract truths. They are plausible, evocative of life in general. They help people make sense of the world. Making sense is itself a fundamental activity in everyday life, bringing order to the world. Events are thematised and made explicable by naming things and events, by describing them in known and familiar ways. Individuals make sense of being healthy or ill by naming relevant events in their lives (e.g. the birth of a baby, an accident at work, the discovery of cancer), which they take to be illustrative of their present state. Of course, different people can and do choose different stories as illustrations but beneath these differences lies the same general principle, that of providing a plausible account of their health and illness.

By making sense, people can also account for the phenomena under consideration. They can assign causality, an attribution which may have little to do with scientific causation or veracity but which demonstrates to the individual why life is like it is. Sense can be made of life by providing general accounts of the 'what happened to me' or 'life is like that' sort. Events are 'explained', therefore, in terms of fate or resignation or individual circumstances and responsibility. Part of the cause of events may also be seen in the context of those events. With health, this context may lead to people recounting stories of work, neighbourhood, and such behaviour as smoking and diet. And if people are uncertain of their place in the world, they may range widely. In a world of apparent constant change, the search for sense may become anxious and wide ranging to include the nature of society itself. In this search, individuals may have recourse to what Bauman calls their historical memory,(34) a group's conception of the past which is not necessarily consciously recognised by that group; for example Britain's imperial past which may engender racist explanations to make sense of world (see Chapter 4).

If people (social scientists and doctors included) make sense of the world through telling stories, how do we (social scientists as social scientists) make sense of this making sense? To explain how we think it comes about, it is necessary turn briefly to social philosophy and the work of the sociological phenomenologist, Schutz.(35) He suggests that there exist in the world several 'provinces of meaning' or 'realities'. The world of everyday life - of everyday occurrences and thoughts - is the most important or 'paramount' reality. In this reality, individuals order and categorise the world to endow it with meaning. Schutz calls these orderings typifications or constructs of the first degree. The 'world of scientific theory' is another province of meaning, one in which clarity, coherence and consistency are important. This compares with the paramount reality which is often unclear and inconsistent. How can the scientist form consistent 'objective' meaning from inconsistent subjective meanings?

The answer lies in the scientist constructing, for scientific purposes, typification of the typifications her/his subject makes in the world of everyday life. In other words, the scientist builds ideal-types or constructs of the second degree. This 'artificial device' provides a likeness of paramount reality, a model of the life-world. "The model, however is not peopled with human beings in their full humanity, but with puppets, with types; they are constructed as though they could perform working actions and reactions...(These) are only assigned to the puppets by the grace of the scientist".(36) Such applies to the scientist's categorisations and typifications and not to individuals in the life-world itself. But the use of the term 'puppet' points to Schutz's view that social science should be observational rather than interactive. The social scientist observes her/his subjects in reference to her/his typology, checking observations with types and typology against observations.(37) And through her/his observations and interpretations, the social scientist can offer a different (not necessarily privileged view of the social world, the adequacy of this view depending on the salience of second-order constructs to the paramount reality, the establishment of the logical relations between characteristics and the valid specification of the context through theoretical constructs (ideal types). In other words, this test of adequacy is a way of ensuring that the interpretations are valid ones. So for interpretative social science to be valid, scientific constructs must, rather than just be amenable to statistical testing, accord with the postulates of adequacy (the investigated individual must be able to understand that which is indicated by the construct), of logical consistency (phenomena must be logically interrelated to one another and to their wider context) and of subjective interpretation (the model or theory constructed by the scientist must use the investigated individual's ideas to account for the facts observed). In general terms, it is a test of the plausibility of the constructs and explanation. So we make sense as scientists in similar ways to those in which individuals make sense of the world in which they live. Part of our test lies with the reader. If we have made sense of making sense then our descriptions, categorisations and explanations will ring 'true'. Again just as with making sense in everyday life, people in our account do not speak for themselves. They have to be named and causality assigned in the name of some general principle(s). We try to let our informants - and they are essentially that, inducting us and providing us with knowledge - 'speak for themselves' by quoting them at length and in their own words to let their stories stand out. But we cannot present all our data and we readily admit that we select those which tell our story best. As will be seen, however, we do point to the apparently contradictory nature of individual accounts and of different individuals in relation to phenomena. Smoking is both good and bad. Industry near a neighbourhood provides jobs close by and pollution to affect health and everyday life. In the end, it is on the plausibility of our story in the light of the three postulates (adequacy, logical consistency, subjective interpretation) that our case rests. We are successful if we have made sense of making sense.

THE STUDY

The ethnographic material on which this book is based comes from an ESRC project looking at regional variations in lay perceptions of health and in the utilisation of health services (data gathered 1985-6) and Donovan's Ph.D. thesis (data gathered 1983-4). The ESRC project involved interviewing between thirty and fifty people drawn from the electoral register of three wards in different parts of Britain: West Yorkshire, East London and the West Midlands. The wards were selected because they had large proportions living in public housing estates, a low proportion with black heads of household, and a high percentage having 'working class' manual occupations. It is precisely people with such characteristics who tend to be more likely to experience health disadvantage, poor access to care in relation to needs and deleterious life-style and habits (Chapter 1). To preserve the anonymity of the respondents, we have re-named the areas and individuals. Fifty come from West Yorkshire ('Deanswood' and referred to as (DW) in this and later chapters), thirty from East London ('Parkheath' (PH)) and thirty from the West Midlands ('Mossley Green' (MG)). Donovan's Ph.D. thesis provides a sample of people of Asian (AS) and Afro-Caribbean (AC) descent living in North and East London. They were not selected form the electoral register because of the difficulties of identifying black people, but from the more informal strategy of snowball and key informant sampling.(38) Thirty people were interviewed - 16 of Afro-Caribbean descent (six men and ten women) and 14 of Asian descent (women only). Those data have been in part re-analysed for this book.

'Deanswood' is a fairly isolated suburb in the West Yorkshire metropolitan area surrounded by major roads and motorways. The ward consists of two distinct parts. One is 'old' or 'rough' Deanswood, a large pre-1914 public housing estate of red-brick terraced and semi-detached houses. The other comprises newer public and private housing developments of mixed designs. There are some dis-used coal mines, and industrial developments on the fringes of the ward, but it is largely residential in character. Of the fifty interviewed, 26 were women, 21 were in paid employment, 6 unemployed and 32 fall into the 35-64 years age-group (39). This is a fairly good mix, although slightly under-represents the unemployed according to the 1981 census, although as we have argued such representativeness is relatively unimportant in our study.

'Parkheath' is a more homogeneous area, consisting of one extensive public housing development to the east of London. The houses were built between the wars and are of red-brick, terraced and semi-detached design. As a result of the 1980 Housing Act, tenants have the right to buy council houses, and approximately one-third of Parkheath residents have chosen to buy and develop their homes. There is now a visible, sharp division between those with and without the necessary means: those who have bought their homes have added pebble-dashing, new doors, new windows or double glazing and central heating; those without are living in unmodernised, deteriorating houses. The area is dominated by a large car-plant, and there are other industrial concerns lining the opposite side of the trunk road to central London. Of the thirty interviewed, 14 were women, 16 in paid employment, 3 unemployed, and 21 fell into the 35 to 64 years age-group. Again, this is a fairly balanced group, although it slightly under-represents the unemployed and elderly.(40)

'Mossley Green' is a mixed area of industrial and residential uses in the West Midlands metropolitan area. The residential development consists of several different estates of varying ages, mostly public housing and comprising old red-brick, newer brick and breeze-block terraces and semis, as well as several low-rise(three storey) flats, tower blocks (fifteen storeys) and two roads of private, detached houses. There is evidence of an old colliery with huge slag-heaps remaining and there are many industrial buildings, most of which housed now-closed smelter and leather works. Like Deanswood, it would appear that very few houses have been purchased from the council. Of the thirty interviewed, 17 were women, 16 in paid employment, five unemployed and 19 fell into the 35 to 64 years age-group. This is fairly representative of the area.(41)

The areas and groups were thus chosen to focus upon the least healthy in Britain - those who have manual occupations and live in public housing. The three metropolitan areas were chosen in order to examine regional variations in perceptions of health and views about health and services because 'the region' has been isolated as the tier for resource-allocation and decision-making. We take the view, therefore, that there may develop a 'regional consciousness', developed and nurtured by the industrial, political, social and communications structures in particular places, which may affect how people think and act. We are all aware of the stereo-typical individuals of Yorkshire, scotland and the Home Counties. We do not know if such consciousnesses exist, how best to tap them if they do, and what effect on thought and action they might have. It seemed worth trying to find out. We shall return then to policy (and method) in Chapter 7 and we now turn to lay beliefs and initially to perceptions of health and illness.

'I COULDN'T AFFORD TO BE ILL': PEOPLE'S PERCEPTIONS OF HEALTH AND ILLNESS

Everyone has an opinion about their state of health. For most, being and feeling healthy is unsurprisingly important, but 'health' itself is difficult to define. Delores believes health exists only in a whole, natural body:

Delores (AC): Once the body is tampered with, something is taken away, that body can't never be the same. The slightest thing can trigger off something somewhere else. People that grow old and have all of their teeth and have everything intact, that's what you would call a <u>healthy</u> body... A natural body, that's the best. Once something is taken away from the body, it's not the same again.

But for most, being healthy is assumed to mean that an individual probably has 'ordinary' or 'everyday' illnesses such as coughs, colds and minor injuries. Health is, by and large, taken-for-granted:

Maureen (DW): I don't think about it (my health) really, until I get a pain... What can you think about your health? I think about going to shop and work, but you don't think about your health.

Gareth (PH): You take it (your health) for granted at 20, and gradually, you think, "Well, I'm in the middle age now and it's a bit more important"... It is not taken so much for granted so it is something to be worked at.

Many share Gareth's view that a person's state of health varies with age. Some remember their childhoods as very healthy times, but accept that increasing age will mean deteriorating health:

Audrey (PH): I'm getting old and I can't do things now that I could do when I was younger, but that doesn't mean to say I'm ill, it's just your bones and muscles seem to get worn out.

Marje (DW): You've got to be badly sometime in your life. When you get to an age you get ill, don't you?

Rani (AS): When you are young you are much better, but as you age, with the time, you get certain illnesses and pains and aches.

Delores (AC): You start OK, but then you go down... I haven't been, like, very ill in my life, but I haven't had perfect health. Everyone gets something.

We will return to the inevitability of illness later. Health and illness are so inextricably related that it is extremely difficult to consider them as separate entities. Health is, however, of particular importance to some. Women with children are an obvious example:

Millie (AC): If I'm not healthy, I've got no-one to look after the kids.

Wendy (MG): Yes, my health is important because if I am ill, I can't cope with Michael (her son) because he is Down's Syndrome.

Alison (DW): When you've got a family - more so when you've got children to look after. You can't afford to be poorly then. No matter how ill you are, you've still got to get up and go... If I felt ill, I'd have to be really ill to go to bed. Really ill.

Alix (MG): [My health] is important to me in one way. Like keeping up with the baby. When I feel down, I can't expect him to go to bed or anything. He needs attention all the time.

James has a dependent, 39 year-old mentally and physically handicapped daughter:

James (DW): I couldn't afford to be ill at all, not with Carol to look after... I wouldn't be able to drive her home from the hospital or anything.

For those without the burden of dependants, health is essential for everyday functions such as work, happiness, life itself:

Steve (MG): Well, I just keep going on. I don't worry about [my health] too much.

Joe (AC): Health is very important. I like workin'. If you're sick, you can't work.

Sufiya (AS): You are only happy when you are healthy. If you are ill, nothing looks good to you.

Leslie (PH): [Your health] is important. I mean, if I was ill tomorrow, then I've got problems.

Albert (DW): Without your health, you might as well not be here because if you're not healthy, you can't get about and enjoy yourself.

For those of Asian descent, their perception of health is informed by their traditional theory of the importance of balance of 'hot' and 'cold' forces in the body. An individual's temperature is seen as being an important aspect of their health. A normal temperature signals health and any deviation from this is seen to be indicative of some sort of illness. Although these ideas have been partly eroded by Western influences, some respondents still fall back on them to make sense of health and illness. So Rajinda refers to a symptom of typhoid as being a high temperature; Reena recalls her headaches are "like a burning sensation in her head"; and Nassem says that measles is "a very hot disease". It can make the children very ill, the temperature is very high", and consequently, "they can't each chicken, meat, eggs and so on because they are very hot foods". We will return to this theme in Chapter 5. These ideas are, however, reinforced by the cold British climate:

Shobha (AS): Sometimes the weather suddenly gets cold and

you get pains and aches in the body; sometimes it gets suddenly hot, and that can cause illness too.

Rani (AS): When they go from one place to another they get tummy upsets, diarrhoea, because the climate has changed, the water has changed... Here the weather, the dampness, the lack of sunshine, it gives you aches and pains in the body. In warm climate, like Pakistan, you do sometimes get illness like cholera, sometimes malaria due to the mosquito.

Tasneem (AS): The climate attacks your bones and you get aches and pains in your body more than at home.

Tasneem relates health and illness not only to climate but to estrangement, being in a strange land, and these views are echoed by some of the Afro-Caribbean respondents (see also Chapters 4 and 5):

Carlton (AC): I had [perfect health] when I was younger. I haven't got it now. It happen to you in this country. I don't think you can get perfect health over here.

Those of Asian descent also perceive some illness to be, partly, the result of disturbance in the natural balance of hot and cold. Feeling ill may, then, often be described as a "burning sensation" (Reena) or a high temperature.

Health is, then, rather a nebulous, unspecific item in people's lives. It is a residual condition, more often than not seen in relation to illness or to the loss of certain abilities and sense of well-being. Illness is much more easy for people to comprehend because it clearly intervenes in their normal lives, disrupting routines and causing difficulties:

Mary (DW): Once I got arthritis, I can't go a lot of the detailed things that we used to do. That has stopped part of my pleasure.

Rani (AS): If you have got pain in the body, you will not be able to perform your duties as you were usually doing. So, whenever you have any sort of ailment, that would be called illness.

Eleanor (MG): things that do get in the way of your life, like serious illnesses. Having cancer or depression.

Leslie (PH): When I can't get out of bed and go to work. That's an illness. That's when I am ill. You cope with anything. You've got to. But when I can't look after my wife and kids, that's when I'm in trouble. I'm ill.

Many people, like Leslie, make the distinction between 'ordinary' illness which can be put up with, and 'real' illness which tends to refer to specific conditions which acquire the label 'serious' and may necessitate seeking professional help:

Pat (DW): Something really serious in that you definitely would call the doctor out for. That, to me, is an illness. A cough or cold and 24 hour 'flu isn't an illness to me.

Claire (PH): Aches and pains, I don't class them as illness. Period pain is not an illness. When you get a long-term thing like bronchitis - serious. I class when you're carted of to hospital and you're in there for a long term - you are ill. Don't really class a little 'flu as an illness.

Miriam (MG): If you have to go to hospital, like, something you have to have an operation or something like that. That's what I think is an illness. If you have got a little ache or pain, I don't think that is illness - it's something you have got to accept when you're getting older.

Delores (AC): When you are a bed patient. That's an illness, say a heavy illness... Only time I was really ill was when I had my hysterectomy.

Nassem (AS): You feel tired, don't feel like doing any work. Sometimes you feel like you are getting a temperature. You will feel shivery or cold... or pain in the chest. These kind of things tell you that you are not very well - are ill.

Frank (PH): I suppose cancer or muscular distrophy is a real illness because it can't be cured.

Real illness is often associated with 'proper cause', i.e. only seeking medical advice when absolutely necessary and all else has failed (see Chapter 6). The constitution of real illness is variable and includes cancer, heart trouble, arthritis as well as, sometimes, 'flu. The problems may be life-threatening or self-limiting. Like health, illnesses are not necessarily seen in the same ways by all people. Some may consider relatively minor conditions to be important. Others dismiss severe, chronic or debilitating illnesses as insignificant. Most view being healthy as a desirable state and some strive to consider themselves to be healthy by ignoring their own health problems. Being healthy is a social construction - it is a topic rarely out of everyday conversation - and it is negotiated in the light of an individual's perceived needs and personal attributes and circumstances.

Indira (AS): As I grew up I was healthy... I had typhoid when I was 10 years old.

Cathy (MG): My husband is healthy... He had a slipped disc and a growth removed from his chest about seven years ago.

Marian (PH): When you're laid up and you have to go to bed because you can't fight it, that's an illness. When you can get around and still carry on, you don't really call that an illness... [anaemia] I've had that on and off since I was a child. It's something I live with and I don't call it a health problem.

Margaret (DW): I consider things that are crippling diseases like arthritis, cancer and heart trouble I'd call as an illness. I don't class me stomach as an illness. It's there, and I've learned to live with it.

Eleanor (MG): I suppose I must be one of the lucky ones... I don't have many complaints - only me eczema and asthma and I've lived with them, so they're not really problems.

The last three illustrate how people with chronic conditions become so accustomed to their illnesses that they almost forget they have them. Their lives have adjusted to them so well that they are able to regain the status 'healthy'. This view is re-inforced by the more serious conditions they perceive others to suffer from. Indeed, there are some, albeit a small minority, who are deeply affected by long-standing illnesses which are so severe they cannot be ignored or accepted:

Alan (MG): I've been disabled for 6 years... In the morning, I'm in agony, trying to get my breath. Half me life I suffered from fibrositis of the spine... I've got pains in me ankles and thumb and in cold weather, they're terrible.

Arthur (MG): This has done me in the last five years... There's lots of things I can't do now. My son has to do everything for me - and exertion. I try to manage, but I can't... Me grip goes, it's like cramp. The joint sticks and the pain is terrible... [the respiratory trouble] happens anywhere, anywhere. I suddenly [gasp, gasp, gasp] and it gets worse. It frightens me.

Edith (DW): I've got osteo-arthritis badly in the feet and I've got to wear callipers to walk about. Quite easily some days, I could just sit here and not move... But I don't, I get up... because I know that at the bottom of you, you've got to, otherwise you'd just stop altogether... It's up to everybody individually to help themselves. There are some illnesses you can't get over, but there is some you can control.

In Edith's statement, the effect of a long-standing illness is justaposed with individual responsibility and the need or desire to cope with medical problems. Definitions and perceptions of illness are often inseparable from their 'causes' and 'solutions' in people's minds (see Chapters 3 and 5). Nor are these definitions and perceptions constructed in isolation. Individuals reply not only on their state of health, but that of others as well and the demands of factors such as work:

Mona (DW): I felt really ill when I had the 'flu, but I wouldn't have said that it were an <u>illness</u>. And I felt really ill when I had the trouble with my stomach, but that were me own fault having too much bran. I think me kid's is an illness, with the asthma.

John (DW): To me an illness is when you are not at work, when you have to take to your bed... There's many times you get a cold and you carry on working, doing your job and you don't let it get you down.

Delores (AC): If you can work and carry on, well you carry it [the minor illnesses].

Nassem (AS): The doctor told me to have two weeks' complete rest, but I couldn't because I had some guests from Pakistan and I also have my children. I had no help at all, so I had to get up, do the housework.

Although not always explicit and clear, there is a sense running through most of the discussions about health and illness of the inevitability of illness. Health is the desired state, often taken-for-granted, but it is lost when illness strikes and this loss of health is expected at any time. Very few people are able to say that they know anyone who is never ill:

Mark (MG): You can always find something wrong. If it's not one thing or the other. I don't think anybody is ever perfectly fit and healthy.

Gordon (PH): Not anybody's got <u>perfect</u> health: everybody's got a small thing, even if it's only an ache in the finger. There isn't anybody that's go <u>nothing</u> wrong with them at all.

Nassem (AS); You can get ill any time of your life. You can never expect that you will always be healthy. A mishap can happen, any time. You can get ill, you can get some disability by accident, because these things are in God's hands and everybody should expect that they will get ill, any time.

In fact, so inevitable is the incidence of some sort of illness, one should not be at all surprised. It may be a matter of luck or fate or God's will, but there is little an individual can (or should) do:

Martha (AC): I break my leg. There was nothin' I could do about that. Yeah - that was just something that happen... I don't worry over sickness. As it comes, you just suffer it. Illness jus' happens, it's nature.

Gareth (PH): As far as cancer is concerned, I believe that everybody has got it and it could be stress or anything that could trigger it off, so, then again, you are just unlucky, aren't you?

Louise (AC): I don't worry about no sickness because what is written is written. Even when I myself became ill, I never moaned, I never grumbled because we don't buy sickness, it just comes.

Rita (DW): What I have to have, I have to have. Just have to face up to it, won't I?

Maureen (DW): It's a fact of life, getting ill, innit? It's a fact of life... There aren't a lot of point, is there? We're gonna die, and if it's gonna happen, it's gonna happen, innit? There's no point natterin' [worrying], is there?

Emily (AC): It's give and take. When it does happen, one should not feel too disappointed. You have to just take it easy and accept it and try to get over it.

These attempts not to worry, to "face up to it" and "try to get over it" are all part of people's attempt to return to a state of equilibrium when illness strikes them. Illnesses are discounted and ignored, and health becomes secondary because of the need to keep going in the light of the obligations of everyday life. There is the hope that the problem will go away. If it does not, some are able to regain a definition of healthy by becoming accustomed to a complaint, or altering their lives so that it no longer impinges upon their activities or obligations (see above). Some, like Edith and Arthur above, will have to accept that they are seriously ill. The threat of serious, debilitating illness usually lurks at the back of people's minds. Gareth (above) and many others fear the onset of cancer or other conditions such as AIDS, heart trouble, strokes and paralysis. The hope is that they will not affect themselves:

Tansneem (AS): There are many illnesses which we are afraid of, like paralysis, blindness, stroke, cancer... We always pray that God should save us from all of these.

Leroy (AC): Cancer. Everybody's born with it, it just takes something to set it off.

Peter (MG): In ten year's time when I go in and - say I've got lung cancer or owt like that, I'll look back and say, 'Come on, get something done'. But it's my own fault for smoking. I wouldn't worry about it until it's happened. If it happens, it happens. That's the type I am.

This perception of the inevitability of illness, and its control by forces outside an individual's power (such as God, fate) will be considered in more depth in Chapters 3 and 5.

People fear the loss of functional capacity brought on by serious illnesses. They want to be healthy and to be seen to be healthy,an attitude which for some, entails their defining away quite serious, often debilitating chronic conditions. Being healthy, then, is in the mind of the individual. She/he perceives and defines it in such a way that it fits their own personal characteristics and circumstances. We are not suggesting that such perceptions are constructed by individuals in a social vacuum. Their circumstances play a significant part in their negotiation of the meanings of health and illness. Indeed, it is only when an illness is considered to be life-threatening or seriously interrupts normal life that the label illness (real illness) is assigned and accepted. Other illnesses are expected to be ignored or worked through. Being healthy means keeping going despite the inevitability of illness. People make sense of this perceived inevitability by expressing opinions about the sources of ill-health. In other words, as people talk about the meanings of health and illness, they inexorably discuss their 'causes'.

FOOTNOTES

1. J. Cornwell, <u>Hard-earned lives</u>, Tavistock, 1984., 19 On these themes see also R. Dingwall, <u>Aspects of illness</u>, Martin Robertson, 1976.

2. This research comes in fact from both the conservative and radical poles of enquiry. Structural functionalism, which places great emphasis on the benign intervention of medical professionals using scientific knowledge, regards lay beliefs as irrational and unscientific. See, for example, T. Parsons, <u>The social system</u>, Free Press, 1951. Radical, often marxist, ideas stress the ideological role of medicine in helping to maintain the capitalist status quo of exploitation and imperialism. While arguing for the 'victims' (patients, clients), lay ideas are regarded as suspect especially if they suggest medicine is beneficial and want more treatment. See, for example, V. Navarro, <u>Medicine under capitalism</u>, Prodist, 1974.

3. A useful summary of this history is provided in A. Giddens, <u>New rules of sociological method</u>, Hutchinson, 1976, Chapter 1.

4. For example, M. Voysey, <u>A constant burden</u>, R.K.P., 1975.

5. B. Cowie, The cardiac patient's perception of his heart attack, <u>Social Science and Medicine</u> 10, 1976, 87-96.

6. See, for example, M. Blaxter, The causes of disease, <u>Social Sciences and Medicine</u> 17, 1983, 59-69; R. Pill and N.C.H. Stott, Concepts of illness causation and responsibility, <u>Social Science and Medicine</u> 16, 1982, 43-52; R. Fitzgerald, <u>The experience of illness</u>, Tavistock, 1984; R. Williams, Concepts of health, <u>Sociology</u> 17, 1983, 185-205. A recent review has been published by M. Calnan <u>Health and Illness</u>, Tavistock, 1987.

7. A point also well made by Cornwell <u>op cit</u>, 144-5. But see M. Calnan, Lay evaluation of medicine and medical practice, <u>International Journal of Health Services</u> 18, 1988, 311-22 for an explicit statement that people do not view the medical system uncritically.

8. These conflicts are discussed in E. Freidson, Dilemmas in the doctor-patient relationship, in C. Cox and A. Mead (eds.) <u>A sociology of medical practice</u>, Collier-Macmillan, 1974.

9. The medicalisation of everyday life is taken to mean the use of medical ideas, the extension of medical competence and so on over more and more facets of everyday life. See I.K. Zola, Medicine as an institution of social control, <u>Sociological Review</u> 21, 1972, 615-30; I. Illich, <u>Limits to medicine</u>, Penguin, 1977.

10. M. Lock, Models and practice in medicine, <u>Culture,</u>

<u>Medicine and Psychiatry</u> 6, 1982, 261-80.

11. See, A.D. Gaines, Definition and diagnoses, <u>Culture,</u> <u>Medicine and Psychiatry</u> 3, 1979, 381-418.

12. D.W. Blumhagen, Hypertension, <u>Culture, Medicine and</u> <u>Psychiatry</u> 4, 1980, 197-227, I.N. Stevenson, Editorial comment, <u>Social Science and Medicine</u> 14B, 1980, 1.

13. Cornwell <u>op. cit</u>, chapter 5.

14. H. Roberts, <u>The patient patients</u>, Pandora Press, 1985, chapter 5.

15. Blaxter <u>op. cit</u>; Pill and Stott <u>op. cit</u>. See also Calnan 1987 <u>op. cit</u>.

16. M. Blaxter, Self-definition of health status and consulting rates in primary care, <u>Quarterly Journal of Social Affairs</u> 1, 1985, 131-71.

17. Cornwell <u>op. cit</u>, chapter 6.

18. See A.Smith and B. Jacobson (eds.) <u>The nation's health</u> Kings Fund, 1988.

19. Roberts <u>op. cit</u>, chapter 4.

20. Themes also shared by Cornwell <u>op. cit</u>, Roberts <u>op. cit</u>. See also Calnan, 1987, <u>op. cit.</u>

21. See, for example, M. Blaxter and E. Patterson, <u>Mothers and daughters</u>, Heinemann, 1982. On these factors and their relationship with use of facilities see J. Eyles and J. Donovan, <u>Regional variations in perceptions and experiences of health and health care</u>. End of Research Report, ESRC Grant no. G00232140.

22. These scales on health state were developed by Ware and his colleagues. See, for example, J.E. Ware, The effects of acquiescent response set, <u>Medical Care</u> 16, 1978, 327-36 and R. Brook and J.E. Ware, Overview of adult health status measures, <u>Supplement to Medical Care</u> 17(7), 1979, 1-131.

23. Health care satisfaction scales developed by Ware and his colleagues. References as at footnote 22.

24. This health status measure is known as the Nottingham Health Profile. See S. Hunt et al., The Nottingham Health profile, <u>Social Science and Medicine</u> 15A, 1981, 221-9; S.Hunt and J. McEwen, The development of a subjective health indicator, <u>Sociology of Health and Illness</u> 2, 1980, 231-36; S. Hunt et al., <u>Measuring health status</u>, Croom Helm, 1986.

25. See D. Silverman, <u>Qualitative methodology and sociology</u> Gower, 1985.

26. OCPS, <u>The general household survey</u>, HMSO, 1984.

27. As an example, let us assume a five point scale on each statement ranging from strongly agree to strongly disagree which we score from +2 to -2. Further let us assume that there are 10 statements in the series. Both individuals A and B score 0 on the series. At first sight, there appear to have similar attitudes but individual A's total score is made up of individual ones of, say, -1, 0, 0, +1, 0, 0, -1, 0, 0 +1, a person of moderate or little opinion. Individual B's score is made up of -2, -2, +2, -2, 0, +2, +2, -2, +2, 0, a person of strong, but variable opinion. For a full discussion, see J. Eyles, <u>Senses of place</u>, Silverbrook Press, 1985.

28. Mehan argues that such research treats information like a package to be transferred between people, separating the researcher from what then becomes a passive community and assuming a privileged position for that researcher because of the alleged superiority of information gained from scientific approaches. See H. Mehan, <u>Learning lessons: social organisation in the classroom</u>, Harvard UP, 1979, See also Silverman <u>op. cit.</u>

29. Quantitative and interpretative approaches should not be regarded as mutually exclusive and it is important to try to build bridges between them. See also Blaxter, 1985, <u>op. cit.</u>, Silverman <u>op. cit</u>.

30. Quoted in R. Burgess (ed.) <u>Field research</u>, Allen and Unwin, 1982. Interpretative or qualitative methods form a series of different related approaches. See R. Burgess, <u>In the field</u>, Allen and Unwin, 1984; M. Hammersley and P. Atkinson, <u>Ethnography</u>, Tavistock, 1983; Silverman, <u>op. cit</u>.

31. See, for example, F.G.Johnson and C.D. Kaplan Talk-in-the-work, <u>Journal of Pragmatics</u> 4, 1980, 351-65. It must also be recognised that if a researcher becomes a participant observer, she/he may play different roles, depending on the relative levels of participation and observation. See R.L. Gold, Roles in sociological fieldwork, <u>Social Forces</u> 36, 1958, 217-23; H.J. Gans The participant observer as human being, in Burgess (ed.) <u>op. cit</u>.

32. On the nature of the accounts and validation, see J.C. Mitchell, Case and situation analysis, <u>Sociological Review</u> 31, 1983, 187-211.

33. A. Heller, <u>Everyday life</u>, RKP, 1984; A. Heller, <u>A theory of history</u>, RKP, 1983. The idea of telling stories to make sense of life is used by T. Blackwell and J. Seabrook, <u>A world still to win</u>, Faber and Faber, 1985 in their history of the reconstruction of the British working

class. We also use Heller's approach more formally in our detailed analysis of the West Midlands material, J. Eyles and J. Donovan, Making sense of sickness and care, Transactions of the Institute of British Geographers 11, 1986, 415-27.

34. Z. Bauman, Memories of class, RKP, 1982.

35. See, for example, his papers, Commonsense and scientific interpretation of human action and On multiple realities in A. Schutz, Collected papers vol. 1, Nijhoff, 1962.

36. Schutz, On multiple realities, 255.

37. Schutz's work has received much critical attention in social science. See, for example, B. Hindess, Philosophy and the social sciences, Harvester, 1977; and more sympathetically, K. Wolf, Phenomenology and sociology, in T. Bottomore and R. Nisbet (eds.) A history of sociological analysis, Heinemann, 1978.

38. These techniques are among many assigned the label 'non-probability' sampling by Burgess op. cit. In this case, one individual was found from each of the two ethnic groups who became a key informant by providing information and helping the researcher (see Burgess op. cit.). the key informants also suggested others who could be interviewed and these in turn offered their friends and relatives. This is snowball sampling. See J. Donovan, "We don't buy sickness, it just comes", Gower, 1986.

39. OPCS, Ward monitor: West Midlands, HMSO, 1984.

40. OPCS, Ward monitor: Greater London, HMSO, 1984.

41. OPCS, Ward monitor: West Yorkshire, HMSO, 1984.

3 'Why me?': the causes of sickness

This chapter and the next (Living in Britain) are closely related. In the next chapter, we deal with the context to sickness in which the individual is seen in relation to the wider social structure, and so living in Britain is thus viewed as being associated with health as seen as a dimension of the quality of life. This chapter, however, focuses attention on the individual and her/his explicit opinions about the 'causes' of illness. These causes are again very much social and personal constructions, but this does not make them any less real to those who hold them. These 'causes' are used to give meaning, understand and explain ill-health, and as such are linked to the meanings discussed in the previous chapter (chapter 2). In giving causal meaning of ill-health, people help to identify who or what is to blame for sickness and this may, in turn, point towards specific coping strategies. Most of those who accept illness as a 'fact of life' will offer suggestions as to the 'cause' of their complaint.

For some, however, sickness is so inevitable that its cause must be unknown. In this case, people still regard illnesses as having some cause but it cannot be explained, and so the important element becomes to whom do the illnesses happen:

> Millie (AC): Why me? But on the other hand, why not you? You are human, and it can happen to you, it can happen to me.

> Rani (AS): Only thing you can do is take care of yourself. If there is anything that makes you ill, avoid doing that... We can just take care, but it depends on God. You can still get ill, any time.

J: Do you think there is anything you can do to stop getting ill?

Phyllis (DW):   I don't think there is, is there? If you're gonna get it, you'll get it.

Alex (PH):   Sometime in your life, you're gonna be ill with a cold or something, or you're gonna catch 'flu... You're <u>bound</u> to.

Betty (MG):   You can't go through life without illness.

Rani hints at the possible importance of individual responsibility or action in the prevention or cause of sickness. Others emphasise this aspect of personal control, suggesting that what you do may determine whether you remain healthy or become ill:

Carlton (AC):   I usually keep myself very, very fit, so that if anything comes to me, I'm strong enough not to take any notice of it.

Wendy (MG):   I think it's your mind. If you have a clear mind and healthy mind, then you have got a healthy body.

Nassem (AS):   There are some ways where you can help yourself to keep yourself fit and healthy by eating proper food, having good sleep and good rest, but there are certain times when a person can't help for the health at all... so, there are ways where you can keep yourself healthy, but there is no guarantee, you can still get ill sometimes.

Roger (PH):   I think you can take care of yourself and look after yourself and diet properly and all that, but I don't think there's any such thing as perfect health. Something will go wrong.

Tom (DW):   I've always looked after myself. I shouldn't have got to 82 if I hadn't!

Individuals can have some control over their health, then, by accepting responsibility for taking 'proper' precautions over parts of their life-style. Not taking these precautions can have serious consequences:

Earl (AC):   A lot of time [ill health] could be avoided, either pay more attention to all those health warnings and eat the right foods... A lot of trouble comes from not taking good advice.

George (PH):   Some illnesses you can bring on yourself, where people are being silly with themselves. If people looked after themselves, then they should be all right ... Some of my [football] players, they run around and they are sweating and when the game is over, instead of going and having a shower and wipe themselves down, they just get dressed and then straight out. It can't do no good ... It will come out one way or another.

Jack (DW): [people make themselves ill] by self-neglect, such as going out and getting wet through, not taking precautions.

Alan (MG): If they neglect themselves ... Some people just drink, they never think of eating. They don't do any exercise. They're either sitting or lolling about all the while.

Sid (DW): When you go out in this [winter] weather, you want wrapping up. Some of these young 'uns these days walk about with pullover on, with their backs all bare. I should image it will tell on them in time -illness or what-not.

If individuals fail to take the proper precautions, not only may illnesses result, but also the individual can be blamed. Ivy's (AC) husband, for example, suffered from a stomach ulcer because, "he was always drinkin', so he didn't have space for eating, or time".

DIET AND EXERCISE

One of the easiest components of lifestyle to control is the intake of food. Many are concerned about their diets and some, like Ivy and Alan above, believe that what you eat can have important effects on health and levels of illness:

Gordon (PH): There's foods like fatty foods that are detrimental. Well, can bring on stomach complaints which could lead to something else. Food is important - you've got to be careful with it. Over a period of years, you get to know what's good and what isn't.

Tasneem (AS): I think if we can eat good food and stay healthy, in that way we will save money... Food is the most important thing for your health. You should spend more on the food than on any other thing in the house... You can get good immunity by eating good food.

Margaret (DW): I don't eat anything fried. If they [family] have anything fried, I grill mine. Fruit I love, but I can't eat it, it's far too acidy. So there are things I know I have to avoid, and if I eat it, I'll have a complete day of being doubled in two until I've passed it through.

Ian (MG): I like fried stuff and I'm surprised I'm not at the doctor more the amount I eat. I do have a lot of exercise with the dog... so that probably compensates for all the wrong food intake.

As well as diet, exercise is seen as an important and controllable aspect of life-style. Some believe it to be essential for good health:

> Carlton (AC): You gotta keep your body in good condition... or your joints will jus' weaken up.

> Leroy (AC): It's very important to keep your body in good shape... If you look after your body, I think in the long run, you'll be better off than someone who don't.

> Marian (PH): Laying on the floor, legs up for about 10 minutes. It's to keep the stomach muscles toned.

For most, however, specific exercises are not seen to be necessary. Indeed, such activity may well be harmful:

> Martin (MG): It can be bad for your health if it is excessive.

> Anne (DW): I don't think to go out and join a club or go jogging and stuff like that - no way! I think jogging kills you anyway.

Most feel that if it is necessary, they get enough exercise in their daily lives. For those with manual jobs or who work in the home, their everyday activities are sufficient: any more would be a chore:

> Matt (PH): I do enough [exercise] at work. It's a pretty physical job. Even though I'm only driving, when I go out delivering, I have to throw the load off that. [HGV driver]

> Mary (DW): I don't run three miles or play badminton and that but I started from eight o'clock this morning and I've done the house through and all the washing. I think that's exercise, to me. Probably not to the doctor, but to me it is.

> Leslie (PH): It depends. If you're a fitness fanatic, you think exercise is important. I don't think it is. I walk up the shop and I get knackered. I'd sooner jump in the car and go up the shop.

SMOKING AND WORRY

Smoking is also viewed ambivalently. Some believe that those who smoke are responsible for specific bouts of illnesses. They see smoking by themselves and others as being a cause of ill-health:

> Steph (MG): It was making me ill. I was getting nicotine poisoning, so I did stop it, but at the time, everybody smoked and it was the 'in thing'.

> Martin (MG): I used to smoke but can't any more [because of the ulcer]... I feel better when I don't smoke.

Frank (PH): It can't do you any good, can it? Filling your lungs with all that. It's not natural.

Gerald (PH): I used to smoke and when I smoked, I coughed, and when I stopped, I didn't... I can run further. I can run faster, so smoking must be bad for you.

Jane (DW): I used to [smoke] but I've stopped now... I had a right bad chest with it.

Winnie (DW): Joe's uncle died of cancer and what we saw come away was terrible. I said I'd never buy anybody a cigarette again after we saw how he had to suffer. He smoked heavy.

But some redefine or negotiate the meanings of health and hazard because smoking helps them get through everyday life. It makes life liveable and although the hazards may be recognised, they are underplayed. In this evaluation, smoking is more beneficial than harmful:

Delores (AC): I smoke a cigarette or marijuana to soothe. It keep me calm, comfort me... I don't say it's bad for your health because some people that don't smoke suffer with bad health in different ways... Some say it give you cancer, but my mother never smoked and she died of cancer. We don't know what's ruinin' our health.

Peter (MG): I found a reaction when I packed it in. If I had two or three pints, me head was going all the while... To be honest, I think I went really cranky when I packed it up.

Leslie (PH): No, it's a load of propaganda. Rubbish! I've got aunts and uncles and my father that've died of cancer and they've never smoked a fag in their lives. My father did, but my aunts and uncles never did. How can they turn round and say it was smoking? ...You go into the doctor's surgery and if you say, "I'm out of breath". They say, "Do you smoke?" "Yeah" "Pack it up then". It's not a cure. 'Cause you smoke, they think that is the answer, but it's not. I smoke, the wife smokes. I've got four healthy kids.

James (DW): I don't think smoking... in moderation, I can't see it being bad. But I could be proved wrong. Drink's the same. People abuse these things. Everything in moderation, that's sensible.

Anthony (DW): They say cigarettes cause cancer, but I know somebody that's smoked all her life - no sign of cancer when she died. And I know someone who never had a cigarette and died of cancer. It does damage you, does smoking, no doubt about that, but there's still a lot to be said about it.

Claire (PH): I agree [smoking is bad for your health], but circumstances make you smoke - you turn to that packet. It's depression. You know you're ill and it's not doing you any good, but it's a leaning post... It does help... I have managed to cut it down, but not cut it out. I have to have it by the side of me.

Brenda (PH): It's both a habit and a comforter. If I'm worried, I smoke more.

Doreen (PH): I'm a worrier. I worry unnecessarily... If (sons) say this and that is not too good, straight away I light up a cigarette. ...If I ring up anything, or check off the bingo in the paper, I light up. It's silly.

Smoking to alleviate worry may seem silly to Doreen, but she and many others firmly believe that the effects of smoking are less injurious to their health than worry. Worrying is seen by almost everyone as a significant cause of illness. For some, indeed, it is the most important cause:

Shobha (AS): Worries are the worst cause of the illness... Any domestic problem, outside pressure from in-laws, husband or home, any kind of pressure can cause you illness.

Alan (MG): [Worry] definitely makes you worse. When I separated from his [son's] mother, she took him and it put me in Hopwood [local mental hospital] for a while. That's how it affects you.

Ruby (AC): If you are worried a lot and have a lot of things on your mind, anything will come to you. I was worried, and then I was with the sugar [diabetes].

Brenda (PH): I think worry and stress cause ever such a lot of things... I suffer quite a lot with me nerves at times and I do think that leads to other things.

Worry is seen to be the cause of many complaints, physical as well as mental. It may be a direct cause or be a contributor to the development of specific illnesses or episodes:

Tasneem (AS): So many illnesses come on because of the worries. Tension, mental tension - you can't sleep very well with the tension. Then, when that will pass, it will lead to illness, won't it?

Betty (MG): Over 12 months you would be surprised what has gone on concerning me mum [she had both legs amputated], what has come out in me, and I think it is only through the worry and strain.

Alix (MG): Well, when I've been worried about the baby, I have felt down in the dumps and not feeling well at all with headaches and aches and pains. It's when you stop worrying that it goes away by itself.

Martha (AC): Worry do bring on sickness, whatever it is. It's tension and pressure and that, and then your nerves may not be able to take it and then you have a nervous breakdown.

Roger (PH): Worry - a lot of people throw it off and say it's harmless, it doesn't <u>cause</u> anything. But you can worry about something and it can really make you ill. <u>Really</u> make you ill, just worrying.

Maureen (DW): [My stomach trouble is] set off by natterin' [worrying]... It's just something you live with, isn't it? It can go away for months on end, even 12 months, and then all of a sudden, something starts it off. Mostly it's temper. You get yourself to such a pitch, everything tightens up.

Sam (DW): Worrying can cause anything. Like losing your hair. It can cause ulcers, can worrying.

The degree of sympathy offered to a sufferer of worry-induced or-exacerbated illness depends upon a perception of the worry as unnecessary or unavoidable. If worry is thought to be unavoidable, then sympathy is offered. Some people, however, are seen to have brought on an illness by worrying too much or without due or proper cause, and they are not always treated sympathetically:

Cyril (MG): I think the wife's mother is one of them sorts. She can worry herself into it. Say somebody has got the 'flu and they come into the house, she has got all the symptoms.

Gerald (PH): It was a problem - not a pain but a discomfort and then I started to worry about it... It dragged on for two or three weeks and it clicked all of a sudden, so I asked them if they were testing for cancer and all of a sudden instead of feeling good I was feeling ill and you can con yourself.

Miriam (MG): As they get older, they sort of sit around and haven't got enough to occupy their minds and they imagine it is worse than it actually is.

Miriam makes a point echoed by many, that illnesses can be made worse by dwelling on a problem. There is, however, a fine dividing line between illnesses that have been caused by acceptable levels of worry and those that have not. People who make too much of worry risk being labelled hypochondriacs:

Tom (PH): They could have something wrong with them and then think it worse. A lot of people don't go to doctors, do they? They'd rather sit and worry about something and it turns out to be nothing.

Colin (MG): Some people, I think, make more of it than is actually wrong with them. I mean, some people have only got to have a finger ache and they are off work.

Geoff (DW): I think they concoct things up and then genuinely believe that it is actually happening to them. They genuinely feel pain. I think that applies to your hypochondriac, doesn't it? Their mind starts it off and then their bodily function comes into being.

Janet (PH): My brother-in-law, he's a hypochondriac. He always thinks something's wrong. But you can bring them on yourselves through your mind, worry, and that kind of thing.

Des (DW): You can make yourself poorly by sitting and thinking about it ... You worry yourself to death if you're that minded.

For some people, worry is an illness in itself, with physical as well as mental manifestations, and it is almost impossible to overcome:

Michelle (MG): Some people bring things on with worry. When they worry, they make themselves feel ill. Well, I suppose it is an illness, worry, you know, depression... I worry unnecessarily and I know I do and I make myself feel ill... headaches, it's like a sicky, heavy feeling inside because I'm the sort that holds it in, you see.

Joe (AC): A terrible headache... You just keep worrying and feel depressed. You can't really understand what is happening. [Joe also suffered from an ulcer.]

Nassem (AS): Depression and worry can cause more illnesses than any other thing. If you are depressed, tensed up, you will get so many illnesses where the doctor will never find out why they are caused. Your stomach may get upset, your blood pressure will rise, you won't be able to get to sleep with depression... Depression and worry are the worst cause for illness. Nothing can cause you more illness than these two things... Most of the people in Britain and the world, I think, are ill because they are depressed... I sometimes think that I am more depressed than ill.

Worry can be compounded by domestic and work responsibilities which can not be ignored. These responsibilities preclude taking 'proper' precautions and can lead to tiredness or more serious complaints. These feelings were particularly noticeable amongst the black respondents:

Delores (AC): It's your problems that make your body sick - what give you all the aches and pains. You're not relaxed if you've a problem... We have the heavy tasks. We rush to get everyone to work, we rush to work, rush at work. Then when you come home, you've got the washin' or cooking or ironing. It's never ending. Time you finished, you have to got to bed... Then you get a few

hours' rest before you gotta be up again for work...
Tiredness can wear you down.

Ivy (AC): I have suffered with me hypertension - backward
and forward, runnin' from work to work, coping with
children. Most of my workmates are blacks, and we all
seem to suffer from this same hypertension.

Tasneem (AS): I felt a bit weak. First of all I thought
it was too much work... perhaps I was exhausted, but then
they found out I had high blood pressure.

Rani (AS): If you are overtired, if you are tensed up,
you will feel ill.

Earl (AC): Once or twice I've been really run down and
get covered in boils and what have you. It's just your
body's way of tellin' you that you aren't lookin' after
your body properly.

A particular form of depression and dwelling on conditions
that produce anxiety manifests itself amongst those of Asian
descent. There is a tendency to dwell on the loss of their
past life, their difficulties in maintaining communication
with friends and relatives in India and Pakistan, and the
realisation that what has been lost can never be regained:

Nassem (AS): I used to be very depressed, missing my
parents and sister. I still do miss them.

Taresh (AS): We feel depressed when we think of our
parents and so on in Pakistan, and sometimes we cry when
we miss them and when we see there is no-one around here
close to us.

Shobha (AS): It can cause a lot of illness. You feel
depressed, you feel unhappy. Since I lost my parents, I
feel like this... I feel very depressed sometimes,
especially when I am alone... Now I feel lonely and that
makes me feel ill and depressed sometimes.

Rani (AS): Loneliness is the worst thing which can cause
illness. If you are sitting on your own, you are all the
time thinking about things. You have nobody to talk to.
If you are with someone, you are speaking, you are just
telling what is in your heart and so you don't feel ill,
you feel happy. But if you are alone, then you will
always feel sick. In our country, people are meeting each
other all the time and they are coming and asking how you
are and that helps lot with your health.

LUCK

Another 'cause' of illness is seen to be luck or chance. Luck
may determine your chances of being healthy or ill, but it is
not, however, seen in isolation. Some link luck with
fatalism, to illness being a fact of life (see chapter 2),

while others believe that luck can be shaped or influenced. The dominant view, that illness is inevitable, seems to correspond with the view that many illnesses have unknown causes. Chance, luck and fate are merely ways of explaining and making sense of things beyond people's knowledge and control. People tend to see themselves as lucky or unlucky in their health compared to others:

Gordon (PH): Well, I don't know, it seems weird. Some people, the whole family has all the complaints you can think of and other people seem clear of it... You can't put it down to clean living because you don't know the circumstances there... At work, there seemed to be blokes going down with all manner of complaints. As soon as they got over one, they were back on it again. I dunno, they must be very unlucky... It seems that some people are a lot more unfortunate with complaints than others.

Janet (PH): We've been healthy. See we think we've been lucky compared to some people.

Earl (AC): Legionnaire's disease... it could affect one person and sort of totally miss another. It's a question of fate.

Mary (DW): You hear some people get all the illnesses, and my friends, three or four of them haven't been in hospital and yet I've been in for six or seven operations, so I've had their share as well. They've just fortunate that they've been lucky in that way.

Gareth (PH): As far as cancer is concerned, I believe that everybody has got it and it could be stress or anything that could trigger it off. So, then again, you are just unlucky, aren't you?

James (DW): Your health is something you are given. It's like plants - you get a strong plant, you can plant it outside. Another, you must treat it with care. I'm very fortunate. A lot of people don't know how fortunate they are.

Good health is sometimes seen as 'running in families', and this may be linked with luck or fate:

Richard (DW): My grandmother, she's about 85 and still going strong. She's had ten kids, too. She's just lucky. You are or you aren't.

Leslie (PH): Not lucky, just the way of life, innit? I mean, we've never abused ourselves. We're all healthy. It's just the way you're brought up... [Illness] is just fate. It's not luck, it's fate.

HEREDITY

The inevitability of illness is also seen in the context of
families.   Many   believe   that   some   conditions   may   be
hereditary, and that they are powerless to prevent themselves
conforming to this pattern:

> Leroy (AC): Cancer. That might be passed down through
> the generations... My mum's mum died of cancer, so my mum
> could catch it, but I don't like to think about that.

> Claire (PH): To refer back to [my family], my grandfather
> died of consumption - that's TB. My father, he had
> chronic bronchitis throughout most of his life. Now it
> seems I've got the chronic bronchitis and trouble with the
> chest, so I do think, yeah, there are things... that go
> through a family.

> Jane (DW): Ulcers - me mam had one, then me dad had it,
> and I'm just hoping I don't get one.

> Dalee (AS): My father's whole family was diabetic, so
> they were careful about the sugar... Ate special things.

> Kate (MG): I think migraine. Me mum gets migraine and
> I do sometimes as well.

> Wendy (MG): My father is slightly diabetic... My
> father's nan was diabetic and on insulin like my daughter,
> so, yes, things like diabetes sometimes can run in the
> family.

Like Wendy, many others thinks that they can see patterns of
illnesses running through their families, but are unsure as
to how or whether it is actually true for their families or
gender:

> Carlton (AC): I know there's a heritage from the father
> to the son and the son to his son... I think there's good
> possibilities of that, 'cause what I've been told about
> my family past... There's been a cycle, like, especially
> for the women. The women, they die, they seem to die very
> early, especially on my mother's side, about 50-55. Like
> they get something inside them. But for me, for the guys,
> I think that the guys usually live pretty long in my
> family.

> Doreen (PH): Me dad and his two brothers all died of
> cancer... Me father had one job, they reckoned it was all
> the gases and things that could have set up his cancer of
> the lungs... the uncle was a welder and the other uncle
> was a chain-maker for ships. But whether it was due to
> the effects of the work, I don't know... Mother had
> stomach cancer as well. I'm sure that was due to her -
> she loved a bit of fat... I think she dug her grave with
> her own teeth. All that animal fat.

Ian (MG): I know some families are susceptible to heart attacks and heart disease. You know, you often hear people say, 'Oh, me brother's had that and so-and-so's got it'. I don't known whether it's true or not.

Pat (DW): Heart disease, I think can be hereditary. My husband's got heart disease, but he's in perfect health at the moment... but his grandmother had heart disease and his mother and his sister all had heart disease, so I think it can be hereditary. Sometimes I think cancer can be hereditary too, but I'm undecided at the moment.

Delores (AC): I can't say what illness runs because my father is 77 and he's still working on his farm. We have no serious illness in the family what I know of.

In the section above, two members of the same family (Delores and Carlton) have different views about heredity as a cause of illness. Like Delores, many people prefer not to consider that illnesses can run through their families because of the fear that disabling or serious conditions may affect themselves or those they are close to. It is always better to hope that the worst conditions strike randomly. Indeed, the doubts that people have over the importance of heredity are linked to the random inevitability of illness and the influence of chance or fate:

Rani (AS): It is not necessary that because the parent has got some illness that the children should get it necessarily, but there are some chances.

Leslie (PH): My dad was ill for years and my brother is going the same way, but, then again, there's another brother and he is as fit and older than me, so, you know. On the other hand I had a sister that died when she was 37 for no reason. So I can't see that it runs in the family. It's just fate.

Mary (DW): Me mum and me father had rheumatic fever and me brother had rheumatics. I think it comes in the family.

J. (Interviewer): Is there anything you can do to stop your children getting it?

Mary: No, What will be , will be... When they ask me, 'Will we get it?' I just have to say, 'Well, You've got to hope you don't. It might miss'.

So far, we have examined views on causes of illness which, depending on circumstances, may or may not be influenced in some way by the individuals concerned. These causes fall within what might be termed people's personal worlds - they can be affected by individual action or lie within the family where they can be accepted and understood. There are, however, other causes of illness, the effects of which are also variable, but which are seen as being beyond the control of particular individuals. They are seen to emanate from the larger physical and social worlds, but impinge directly and explicitly on individual lives. They are elements of the outside world which possess the greatest immediacy because of the nature of their impacts on people's everyday lives. 'Germs' and the 'environment' are the clearest examples of these 'external' factors.

GERMS AND THE ENVIRONMENT

By 'germs' the respondents mean bacteria, viruses and all other micro-organisms which are simply there, part of the environment and part of everyday life. As they cannot be seen and do not always conform to expected patterns or rules, they are viewed somewhat fatalistically:

Dennis (DW): You've got to be ill sometime. I've never known a person not be ill... Even with a cold, or you catch 'flu - it's just one of those things.

Leroy (AC): I seem to get a cold once a year. Just germs travelling around in the air... this bad 'flu they say comes from Japan. It's in the air, there. You can't help catching it.

Rani (AS): There are many illnesses caused by the germs. The 'flu - one person can catch the 'flu from the other... TB is a very contagious disease which is spread out due to the germs... Also smallpox and measles.

Carlton (AC): I just catch [the 'flu] from a friend or being in the wrong place at the wrong time... the body's overheating, like there's something inside the body working overtime... Something your body's fighting against.

Delores (AC): When you get coughs and colds - that's germs. Especially when they get under the skin where you can't see them. Then it get sort of bacteria or inflammation.

But people do not succumb to the influence of germs all the time. Although their ability to cause the illness is viewed somewhat fatalistically, most people believe that the body has a natural resistance which can protect it from germs. An individual may be able to build up this resistance, but, sometimes, germs will overcome it and the individual will become ill:

Gerald (PH): You are susceptible to everything... If a serious bug comes round, no matter what good health you're in, there is still a chance of you getting it. You may have a better chance than others if you are healthy, but you are not immune.

Earl (AC): [germs] are here with us all the time. It's just our body resistance goes up and down... Dependin' on how much you look after your body, your resistance to those germs will fluctuate.

Emily (AC): It is the white blood cells that fight the germs in the body, so if the white blood cells is low, then when the germ gets in the body, it is very difficult to fight it. [She is a trained midwife and so offers a 'medical' version.]

Tanseem (AS): If you are healthy and you have got good immunity, then you will be less attacked by the germs. Then if you are a weak person, you will be more attacked by the germs and quickly you will catch the disease from another person.

Rani (AS): Germs are the cause of illness, and to avoid the germs, cleanliness is the best thing... Cleanliness and freshness [of food].

Delores (AC): I cannot resist colds, just like your body cannot resist everything... The children all had chickenpox and I nursed them and I didn't get that. So it's the sort of thing that the body can resist. But what really is it? What cause it?

Germs, then, are disease-carrying agents and an integral part of the environment. This larger environment is also seen to cause illness less directly. In these terms, the environment is broadly defined and may include aspects of neighbourhood, climate, urban living, housing and pollution. Of these, climate is of particular importance to those who have lived in warmer parts of the world:

Donna (AC): In this country, as you get older, your health really suffers, but like old people in warmer countries like Barbados, you can't tell someone's age, but here, in England, you look older before your time. I think mostly it's to do with the cold weather: as you get older, you feel it and things get harder for you. In warm countries it's just not like that - no rheumatic pain and stuff... So many older people suffer here from cold weather. If they could just live in the warm sunshine they'd be all right - well, they wouldn't be cured, but they'd be better off.

Carlton (AC): Now I see that my own parents might start to have rheumatism which is not really right for coloured people... So that's definitely telling me that I will have it if I stay here too long. Nobody in Barbados suffers from rheumatism.

Indira (AS): The dampness and coldness in this country. We don't get enough sunshine in this country and we get aches and pains in the whole body.

Rani (AS): The sunshine in our country [Pakistan] makes you perspire a lot and that makes you feel better... In this country... you don't have that and you don't feel so good as you do in your own country. In our country, you can get fresh air all the time, but here you have to keep all the doors and windows closed to keep out the cold weather and this affects your health too.

Some people feel trapped by urban living and would like to move away, often influenced by memories of a rural past:

Gerald (PH): I don't like the industrial area. I prefer the country area, but there it is, I am stuck with this and this is all I can afford right now. If I could afford it I would move.

Leroy (AC): Living in London! If you were out in the country, you'd breathe all the fresh air and all that lot. It might not matter a great deal, but livin' in this sort of area with all these cars and chimneys and all that, you can get lead disease.

Shiela (PH): I don't mind it here, but I'd rather go back to 'Southfield' - there's more fields, it's more open.

Some people, like those above, remember a past that was full of health. In some cases, the unpleasant present is compared nostalgically with an idealised version of the past which cannot be regained, even if it existed. There is another group, however, who see the present as healthy and remember a very unhealthy and environmentally unpleasant past. Sickness, for these, was often caused by poor living conditions in the past. Indeed, 'Deanswood' and 'Mossley Green' were public housing estates built to house those removed from slum areas which were completely destroyed. Others were brought to the two areas because they were considered to be good for people suffering from severe chest complaints:

Jack (DW): I were a sickly child... We lived in a flood district, the child mortality were very high. I can remember at least five in my class that died with scarlet fever... Outside there were no dustbins, just used to throw rubbish in a hole in wall... In fact, house were so bad that when they evacuated everybody out and brought us up to Deanswood, they burned them down.

Anthony (DW): I had bronchitis... I suppose it were where we lived. Must've been 'cause we lived in back-to-backs, outside toilet and a lot of fog and smog in those days and a lot of damp in houses.

Nina (DW): We lived in a one-up and one-down, and we had one toilet for three houses... In next street, there weren't water closets, there were linen closets that were emptied once a week and there were no chemicals so you can guess what they were like... It didn't matter what you did or how clean you was, they were built from old wood, it were already infested... When they first moved us to the estate, all your furniture used to be taken in a van to a disinfestation centre and everything had to be disinfested before they'd let you take a corporation house.

Doris (MG): It was always noted as a healthy place... It used to be all fields when we came here. They used to send people with asthma to live round here.

Cathy (MG): We used to get all the fumes and dust and dirt [in the old houses] and then Tracy got asthma and they put me on the list for up here with a better environment, healthier. It's got a park up here, so it has got to be better.

Albert (DW): Up here it is healthy because years ago they moved people up here for health reasons, for chest complaints, bronchitis. What with it being so high up and healthy, woods nearby.

Paul (DW): That's why we moved up here. We lived in 'North Road' and they moved whole family up here because me father was right ill with bronchitis and asthma and they sent him up here because air was better than other side of city. Kill or cure estate it was called!

Of course, the three metropolitan areas are different, environmentally, and so they provoke different conditions and responses. Most people consider Mossley Green and Deanswood to be healthy areas, but this is not the case with the majority from Parkheath. A few react in an acquiescent way to the area, accepting poor environmental conditions perhaps because it is their home:

George (PH): Don't matter where you live, it's only as healthy as you make it.

Susan (PH): It's good as anywhere else, I suppose.

Others, however, are more outspoken and criticise the levels of pollution which, they think, may have an effect on their health:

Lilian (PH): I think Parkheath is an atrocious place... people allow their children to do as they like and destroy things... We have got pollution all around us.

Gerald (PH): The industry causes air pollution. It's something you don't consider as a youngster, but as you creep on, you wonder what it might be doing.

Claire (PH): It's so closed in around here...closed in, dirty, claustrophobic... There's [large industrial plant] down the road. It's very polluted. I don't like it. I must say I'm at the worst end of Parkheath. Definitely. You're on the main road, heavy traffic and the docks further down.

Pollution is also seen as a problem, perhaps a cause of illness, in Deanswood:

> Richard (DW): The air's cleaner down south. It's mucky here... There's lead works up the road. They reckon that's a bit naughty.

> Ron (DW): We've always had that smell from pit... [house builders] built a site down there and now they can't sell them... It's a horrible smell, like sulphur... It got into air and we had to turn all lights off and evacuate once.

> Don (DW): They once called this the anus of the city and I think they were right. Gypsies and there's a trip over there and sometimes it smells bloody terrible. Where Deanswood pit was, where they've built them new houses, you can smell gas, methane...coming from underground workings.

Pollution is noticed by some in Mossley Green, but for those with longer memories, they remember very much higher levels of pollution before the recession of the early 1980s hit the industries of the West Midlands:

> Colin (MG): The smog, it's in the air that you breathe. That makes it bad but it ain't half as bad as it used to be because half the factories have closed down.

> Stuart (MG): People used to say it was polluted, but there aren't so many factories around now.

> Eleanor (MG): Well, when I walk to work in the morning, I don't think it is particularly healthy. I have to walk through the industrial site and there is a white car that has been parked there and it has gone all yellow from the pollution...there's a foundry and you can taste it sometimes, very sweet tasting.

> Steve (MG): It is [healthy] now because all the factories have closed. Over there, you can see 'Arbor' Castle and you couldn't used to see anything through the smoke.

Many respondents narrow their focus to implicate the more immediate environment of housing conditions and neighbourly relations in assessing their states of health. This consideration of the social environment provides and explicit link to the wider social world which is discussed in chapter 4. Living in Britain is the context in which their lives are set. Poor housing particularly is often seen as a cause or exacerbation of illness:

> Lilian (PH): I waited 15 years to have tarmac put on the back... I've got a ceiling that's been black since we've lived here and it's to do with the roof - they have no felt under the tiles, so that when it rains it comes

through and it has gradually spread the black. They [the council] come in and say it's condensation... They put things in the window to let out the steam and that. I had one in the bathroom and it is right over the toilet, it was blowing down your neck... and it was freezing cold... You get all the draughts from the windows... I used to put an umbrella up in me bed because the wind used to blow as if it were outside.

Frances (DW): It's too noisy round here. House is very old - about 80 years and it's damp.

Penelope (PH): The area is damp and the houses are very cold. When you're all out of work, you can't afford a heater.

Alix (MG): There's a fire-bug going on at the moment. They are shoving things through the letter-box and setting fire to the flats... We have got cupboards in the kitchen which are a health hazard... I would rather live in a house where it is safe and away from all this violence and things like that. [She lives in a flat on the second floor of a fifteen-storey tower block.]

In Alix's comments, the effects of housing are related to the social conditions of neighbourhood. These conditions are also seen as causes of ill-health and are often expressed in terms that will recur (eg race, crime) in the next Chapter. Sometimes people also sense a deterioration in conditions over time:

Jim (DW): If I won the pools, I would go and live somewhere else... You get the council shoving problem families on your doorstep.

Marian (MG): Well, there's quite a lot of blacks moving in now and scruffy people. It used to be nice and posh.

Alec (PH): Years ago, you didn't shut your street door. The neighbours would come in and borrow this and that. Never a bolt on the door. You trusted everyone. Today, you put locks, bolts on when you go to bed.

CONCLUSION

People's accounts of what causes sickness, then, are social constructions which are negotiated in the context of their everyday lives while taking due regard of individual attributes and circumstances. These causes are not like scientific causation in that they are clearly right or wrong. They may, indeed, be 'wrong' according to medical science but they are still real in their effects because they make sense and are believed. There is a clear division between illness that 'just happens' and that that can be avoided. On some occasions, illnesses strike some and not others without any apparent reason, or just arrive 'out of the blue'. Often the chance of becoming sick is seen to be dependent upon luck or fate. On other occasions, individuals can be seen to be implicated in the causes of illnesses by doing something which is thought to have contributed to their own health problems. They are then seen to be responsible, to be 'to blame', and then sympathy may not be offered or be withdrawn.

There are, however, no universal criteria that people use to allocate blame to others or themselves, or to decide upon the influence of luck or fate. Life-style, time of year, family and personal circumstances, the pressures and strains of everyday life may conspire to cause ill-health, but it is also true that these characteristics form the context within which cause is itself judged. By acting in both these ways, of effect and form, these characteristics also shape the internal consistency of the accounts people give of the causes of illness. Illnesses are seen to have 'proper' causes, and people's notions of causality are rational. Their theories may differ from scientific causation, but must be regarded as equally rational systems of thought ordered differently. They are not inferior to scientific theories and a very real impact on behaviour and attitude. The rationality of the system is maintained by assigning the label 'hypocondriac' to those with illnesses which are not seen as having due and proper causes.

Some illnesses, however, are considered to be more inevitable, in that individuals can do little about them. 'Proper' cause implies that certain actions can result in more or less illness, but for some conditions the causes are seen to be out of individual control. In these cases, illness is bound to occur and so it is more a matter of whom they strike rather than why. Germs are one of these causes. They are there, invisible and part of the environment everyone has to share. Germs are everywhere and can strike at any time. Differential impact results from luck (being in the wrong place at the wrong time) or levels of resistance (natural, largely, but also to some degree self-made). The environment itself is viewed similarly. It is 'out there', and its effects are imposed on people. In most accounts, people just report how the environment (past and present) has affected or might in the future affect, their health. It is largely beyond their influence, just part of everyday life in Britain.

4 'News is bad': living in Britain

In previous chapters, we have described how people make sense of health and illness, negotiate their definitions and perceptions, and shape their experiences of health and illness mainly in their own (lay) terms. These definitions and perceptions of experiences point to the significance of a sort of fate, acquiescence and sense of powerlessness which are produced by the circumstances of everyday life. These circumstances are not matters of the individual alone. Her/his experience is shaped by wider social forces which we began to discuss in chapter 3. People's experiences cannot be divorced from these forces; indeed, they are embedded in them. They are, however, apparently outside of any individual's control because they are simply part of living in Britain (see also chapter 1). In the discussion that follows, people's experiences of health and illness are seen in terms of life in Britain, which comprises, for them, work, racism, poverty, unemployment, crime, youth and the future. Often these factors are expressed in terms of concerns about 'social change', especially the way things are changing.

WORK

Work is an extremely important factor in people's lives. For those who have jobs, their work is often so important that it is the item against which all others are judged. Illness, for example, may be defined according to whether or not it is incapacitating enough to prevent the individual from working (see chapter 2). Illnesses which can be 'worked off' are not considered to be 'real' illnesses, but just minor inconveniences that are part of life. Where an individual is out of work or does work which is generally seen to have little value and prestige (such as house work), these considerations do not usually hold, and some of these individuals specify more minor complaints and consider these 'illnesses'. The unemployed and house-workers may feel that they possess less social worth than those in paid employment. This perception may, in turn, lead to depression and demoralisation as well as low levels of personal well-being. Two of the unemployed men, for example, revealed that they were suffering from agoraphobia, and others admitted that they suffered from many episodes of ill-health: chronic as well as acute; physical as well as mental or psychological:

> Dennis (DW): Trying to get a job round here, it's near damned impossible. I don't care what anybody says. So many people, and when you say you're over 39, they don't want to know. You're over the hill.

> Louise (AC): When I was workin', I was very happy because when you get up in the morning, you clock your card in and then on a Friday, you have a bit. Now I have to wait on Social Security to give me a penny on which to live.

> Sandra (DW): Unemployment and owt like that, I think it's awful. Well [my husband] has been unemployed for three years. He were good at his job but he is too old now, too old. He could've had jobs but the younger men got them. 55 you are too old.

> Sophia (AC): If I stayed home it would affect my health because I would be bored, stiff bored.

> Alix (MG): It's very hard [both being out of work]. We will just have to try to soldier on as much as we can. I would like a job... [Husband] is looking for a job but there's none about at the moment. It's really hard round here. He's never had a job since he left school.

> Carlton (AC): The whole incentive to do anything was gone... You have so much [anger] in you, if someone was to come at me at the wrong moment, I'm sure I'd just rip their head off their shoulders with my bare hands, you know? The pressure inside just fill me up... I think I was going mad, I used to talk to myself.

> Brenda (PH): [Being out of work makes my husband] more insecure. And they lose a certain amount of self confidence.

Those who are in paid employment, however, do not always escape health hazards. Indeed, among these groups, most of those with jobs had typical manual occupations. Many of these posed specific hazards, either immediately in the form of occupational 'accidents' or more long-term through exposure to harmful conditions which sometimes result in chronic illnesses. These poor and dangerous conditions can be found in all the areas sampled, but it is the black respondents who relate the worst examples:

> Louise (AC): (factory worker) We used to work a lot with chemicals - hairsprays, powders, sun lotions and stuff...

I worked there eight-and-half years, and from then on, I was sick [with cancer of the breast and cervix].

Taresh (AS): (home sewing machinist) I get pain in the eyes and in the muscles in the shoulders because I have to bend for long periods over the machine. [If she works all day, she can earn 10 pounds.]

Carlton (AC): (permanent nights in a factory, before he was made redundant) I know there's things in that place could kill me, or do me harm. I'm not too sure about permanent damage, but I'm sure this could give you damage for years ahead and it can get into your body and if you have children, I know they can come out not how they're supposed to be.

Joe (AC): (shift railway fitter) They didn't worry about asbestos 10 years ago... Now they give us a cotton mask... That asbestos is dangerous, 'cause it can't burn, it just powder up and you might breathe all that in and it stick to your lungs inside and it must affect you... Although we have extractor fans [now], you can actually taste it, feel it going onto your chest.

Judy (AC): (care assistant in an old people's home) [The residents] are really smelly, like the ones that suffer from cancer and Parkinson's. You've got all sorts of things coming out of them and you've got to inhale that when you're changin' them... Sometimes you can feel it breathin' down you.

Frank (PH): (operating theatre orderly) I strained my back once lifting a patient... and that dirty needle I stabbed myself with [necessitating a course of anti-tetanus injections]... I'm looking for another job because the pains in my hands and shoulders get much worse at work.

Peter (MG): (welder) Two busted legs, busted hand - through the job in the tank. One was on the waggon, I got trapped. It was no problem. All they do is pay your wages, but I was off four-and-a-half months.

Arthur (MG): (bus driver/mechanic) I had that accident on my knee and it started off all this trouble [disabling arthritis]... A sledgehammer came off the spring-shaft and hit me. I never claimed compensation... they showed me the knee and hip joints and they were all black shadow where the arthritis is.

Jack (DW): (labourer) I fell about 47 feet... and broke me pelvis. I broke me nose, I smashed that arm, compound fracture in me leg. I fact, they scraped me off the floor and they whipped me to hospital... You can't help it, love, you fall and that's it.

Jack's final remark sums up many people's attitudes to their jobs. Work may cause severe health problems, but even so, it is liked and occupational hazards are 'part of the job'. Having a job was itself seen as being important for social worth, for having a place in society, and for a sense of well-being, despite the risks. Without paid employment, little is worthwhile and nothing can be enjoyed because of financial constraints. Most needed and wanted to work above all else:

Delores (AC): (care assistant at an old people's home) although it might not be good for the health, I enjoy doing it.

Don (DW): (disabled miner) I've been a miner all my life... until I retired with ill-health. I saw the coal board doctor and he examined me and advised me to pack it in. Me heart trouble, you know, and other things... I enjoyed being a miner.

J (interviewer): Do you think it affected your health?

Don (DW): That's worse thing about it, it affects your health. [cough, cough]... I were fit enough until I got this anaemia... I think boring machine made me deaf... Sometimes I get that ringing - tinitis - noises in me ears... It sends you potty. [he also has pernicious anaemia, myxoedema - thyroid trouble, angina and chronic bronchitis].

Alan (MG): I'd sooner be at work if I could. I'd be at work tomorrow if I could. They keep coming for me to go, but I can't do it.

Joyce (PH): (Senior sales assistant) I like giving orders... Ever since I've been back at work I've relaxed a lot more. It's done me good.

Leroy (AC): (scaffolder) You get fresh air, you're moving about all the time. Since I've been there, I feel I'm a bit stronger, I can lift heavy weights. I'm fitter. I think it's doing me good... I enjoy what I do. I'd far rather be at work than at home.

It would seem that work can have a clear influence over people's lives. Risks can be accepted (or ignored) because of the benefits (financial and social) of being in 'gainful employment'. The spectre of unemployment is feared by many and hated by most of those who are out of work. Some, like Sean and his wife (DW) and Alix and her husband (MG) have never experienced being in work. Others, like Dennis and Mick (DW), find that once they get to a certain age and find themselves out of work, they cannot get another job, no matter how hard they try. Some respondents, or members of their families, have been forced to take demotion or unattractive jobs because of the changing nature of employment opportunities:

Brian (DW): Now I work for my cousin. Not out of choice, but out of necessity 'cause I couldn't get a job... The conditions aren't good as what they could be. It's dirty and smelly - poor environment, dirty environment... If I could find a better job I'd... This recession has hit the places that looked after the workers better.

Alison (DW): [My husband was] doing a job that's essential [for the water board]. His job's had to go and so they've put him onto a job that he did 20 years ago, which cut his wages down a heck of a lot and also cut down his pride. To us, he's been thrown to the wolves after 35 years, and then they do that. It makes you pig-sick.

Miriam (MG): [My son] hasn't got a job... He gets very depressed because he has always been used to working, but we find him little jobs to do like outside, painting and decorating. He doesn't do too badly as far as money is concerned; his dad and I help him out, but I think if you live in a family where they haven't a lot of money and he'd got to live on his social security money, that's when they start to get depressed and they start to get off on the wrong road.

The link between unemployment and perceived increasing levels of crime and violence are considered further below.

It is clear, then, that work, or the lack of it, may have pervasive effects on people's sense of social worth and well-being. In this regard, health is seen to be affected in broad terms: it is not simply a matter of physical health, although this too may be important, but it is also how state of mind is influenced. Living in Britain with its range of job opportunities determines people's quality of life which in turn shapes their sense of well being, physically and mentally. When people talked about British society, they usually discussed it in terms of the problems and difficulties which directly affected their everyday lives, and health itself was not always dealt with explicitly.

RACISM

An important aspect of society divides the respondents. Racism and the importance of skin colour are seen in different ways by the black and white respondents. For the blacks, racism is an insidious 'fact of life', something which they have to put up with (although they are not sure as to why), and it affects all parts of their lives, deeply:

Ivy (AC): [racism] is there and you know it's there. You can feel it all the time, everywhere. You know you're black.

Delores (AC): I don't even like to think what the effect is. It can wear people down... It makes you feel bad inside, angry, and then one day it will come out... This racial thing, we will get over it. We have to live through it and be strong. We have to. It's the only way to carry on, to survive.

Carlton (AC): I'm not going somewhere just because of my colour, I'm going as an individual... [Racism's] got to stop somehow. Like unless you stop it, it isn't going to stop. Then people will just fight fire with fire; people will get mash up. You can't stop. Once something's started that's bad, you can only treat it with bad. It has got to get worse before it gets better. It's getting worse.

Leroy (AC): I don't know why we have to go through all this being shown up. It gets me mad and I lash out. That's why I really look forward to my holiday in Barbados. There's no more headaches, no more worries about being at work, going out and getting called names.

Tansneem (AS): Sometimes the boys pass us and they pass some remarks. We know at heart they are not as good as they should be. The others, maybe they have certain grudge about us, but they don't show it so much. They keep it in their hearts, whereas the teenagers, they can't hide it.

Nassem (AS): It affects your mind. If you feel depressed that you are not treated as other people are or they look down on you, you will feel mentally ill, won't you? It will depress you that you are not treated as good as you would be in your own country. So if you are not treated well racially, it will affect your health in some way. It will cause you depression, and the depression will cause the illness. .

Shobha (AS): Some people beat my son at school and broke his finger. After that I gave a report to the police and the school... Mrs. Thatcher says immigrants will swamp the country. The way she talks makes people think we are not good people, but since we came, more jobs are going around. But she keeps on being prejudiced, saying immigrants are spoiling the country, making it dirty. All the things we do for the country and she doesn't take any notice of the work she gets from us.

Donna (AC): The government... they would like the black people to leave... They wanted people to come and do all the dirty jobs, sweep the roads and so on, run the buses - all the jobs the people here didn't want to do. Now that these people have worked over here, had their children, here, why should they be made to leave? Especially if they don't want to go... They've put their labour into this country. I'll never think of this country as my country... But I think it's unfair that people who've made their lives here, worked... to then be forced out of the country... Some people, like mostly a lot of English people, they can't accept that the country's been 'invaded' [ironic tone] by Indians, Blacks, Greeks and

that. They don't like it. Me, I'm not bothered... I'd
be really annoyed if someone said to me, 'Go back to your
own country'. I mean, I don't class this as my country,
but it's where I've been since I was seven... In certain
countries what is black countries like South Africa,
Australia, and now English people have taken over, and you
don't hear an uproar about that... In certain countries,
black people are not allowed to go and yet it's their
country, but run by a white government, and what can you
do? You can say all these things but people don't
understand - 'We just want you out of England' - you
know... There's a lot of people in England think that,
but I just don't let them bother me. I'm just here to
work for myself and I don't care what you think - nothing
you say is going to depress me.

Some of the English people Donna refers to are quoted below.
For some black people the police are a focus of discontent
because of their attitude towards black people which reinforces and brings violence to the already racist climate in
which they have to live:

Carlton (AC): If I saw a policeman dyin', I would want
to walk right over him. In the end, I might stop, think,
'Give the man a hand', but I'd have to think twice. I
know there's some hatred from me which there shouldn't be,
but it's there 'cause of the way the police treat us.

Ruby (AC): The police don't give 'em a chance, the black
kids. They can't get work to do; they can't go up the
street... [After arresting her son, the police came to
Ruby's house] They push me, three of them. They push
me and came through the door, up into his room. They see
nothing and go into my room... They look for money and
they don't find none... I say, 'Get out, is only me here
and I'm a woman, so get out'... Then they tell a lie,
that I was furious, in a rage, taking up things to hit
them, but I never... We can't tell no one who will
believe an old woman like me turn up against three police
and fight them. [My son] was in seven months and no bail.
Then, they give 'im one year [in prison]... A lot of
things on my mind. For my son, if he walking on the
street, the police pick him up an' say he attempts to do
this or that... Those things upsetting me; get me
annoyed, get me upset. So, the quicker way I get out of
this country, the better off I'll be... I can't stand it,
can't stand much more. It get me down, it get me sick.

For the black respondents, then, there is a clear link between
the racism they experience daily and their state of health,
physical and mental. The younger people (Donna, Carlton,
Leroy, Shobha) indicate that they are not willing to let
racist behaviour affect them for much longer. Some can
attempt to ignore racism, but it will not ignore them. As Ivy
points out, the colour of your skin means that prejudice is
always there, "You can feel it all the time", and because of
the attitudes and behaviour of whites, "You know you're

black".

The white respondents seem to have no understanding of the effects of racism. None of them was specifically asked about their views on race or racism, but a significant minority, particularly in 'Parkheath', London, expressed racist opinions spontaneously in response to questions about their health or society in general. Donna's arguments above are diametrically opposed by Leslie and Alec:

> Leslie (PH): I've been unemployed on and off for most of my life. I can remember 10 years ago, I could've left a job in the morning and got one in the afternoon. As simple as that... Going back to your coloured immigrants, they're taking up all the jobs and they [employers] don't want to pay a wage no more, not a good wage. If I walked out to a job tomorrow and it was advertised at 100 pounds a week, I'd go down to the bloke, 'Leave off, mate, that's not enough for me. Not to feed my wife and kids on'. So, they know full well that an immigrant or a coloured fellow going to walk into that job afterwards and think it's the world. 100 pounds is the world. And they'll take it and do the job which I've refused to do. It all started with London Transport. That's what started this immigrant thing. They advertised abroad for people on the buses 'cause no white people would do it because it was unsocial hours. That started it all off. All your dirty jobs. They'd take them now, course they would, because the wages would have to go higher. They've got to pay someone. Same as the dustmen. Years ago, no-one wanted to pick up a bin. Now, you can't get on that firm, now. Not for love or money. 'Cause the wages are astronomical. You don't see many coloured doing it.

> Alec (PH): It used to be nice down Hackney Wick, but now it's like you're in Mombassa or something. There's thousands of coloureds. Too many, I think. The government did wrong letting all of them in. Too many. That's what started this country going down. You didn't hear of no drug addiction before they all come over, did you?

Racist views are also expressed in other areas, some about black doctors:

> Colin (MG): I think they need a new hospital because everybody that I have spoken to says that all these beds have been full and they are nearly all blacks what's in the beds.

> J (interviewer): Do you think this is a healthy area to live in?

> Maria (MG): No... Well, there's quite a lot of blacks moving in up here now and scruffy people, so - It used to be nice and posh, but...

Gordon (PH): On the rare occasion I go [to the surgery], I'm not satisfied, no. I don't know whether it's because I can't stand darkies, but, to me, he doesn't have the appearance or know-how of what's going on. He just doesn't fill me with confidence.

Susan (PH): I don't like [the doctor's] attitude. I think it's his face - he's got a permanent grin on his face... I don't understand half of what he says, anyway. He speaks very quick and he is Indian or Pakistani.

Leslie's opinions have been quoted at some length before, but he goes on to express more virulent racist beliefs in his explanation of why life is like it is. Again it is important to remember that his expressions were spontaneous and uninvited:

Leslie (PH): I am colour prejudiced. 100%. I don't like them. I don't let myself get experience with them, you see. I don't like them. I don't like working with them. I don't like talking to them. I just don't like them. As far as I'm concerned half of them only got over here because we owned the British Empire. It should never have come about. It's everybody to their own kind. The should all go back to their sunny countries and then there wouldn't be a housing problem in this country today. And there wouldn't be a work problem, neither. Simple as that... I don't know why you're asking me all these questions about my health. There's nothing wrong with my health, it's the wogs that are the problem.

CHANGING BRITISH SOCIETY

Race is, then, an important aspect of living in Britain. For blacks, it is a depressing, demoralising force which affects them throughout their lives. It causes anger and frustration because it is inexplicable and pervasive, and has effects on black people's physical health and sense of well-being. For the whites, race is an easy explanation for their own social problems. Blacks become the scapegoat for poor housing and high rates of unemployment. The Tory government's place in re-inforcing these attitudes had not gone unnoticed by several. But race is not the only aspect of social change that is noted by the respondents. There is a general sense that 'things are getting worse', that there is a worsening in people's sense of well-being. Quality of life and hence health are seriously affected. In producing anxieties and worries, crime and violence, unemployment, poverty, youths and hooligans and present government policies loom large. Society is seen to be changing for the worst:

Gordon (PH): I think the society we're living in is a lot worse than it used to be. We can remember living here when you could leave your front door open... no-one thought of locking everywhere up and having guard dogs. Society used to be a lot better then. People were better to one another. I can't remember a time when there were so many muggings, women getting raped... Crime and that sort of thing is on the uptake more and more.

Paul (DW): All these muggings and this kind of thing, it's the way kids have been brought up... Young fellows who get caught, I don't think the penalties are hard enough... Treat violence with violence. I've always believed in that.

Brenda (PH): I can't understand why it's changing like it is. I don't like the violence and all the muggings and the selfishness in people. They're all for themselves all the time. I don't like that attitude.

Winnie (DW): I don't know what to think about all the violence. It's beyond me that they seek after that rather than be friends with one another. There's more going on now in the way of muggings than we've ever heard before and less people going to church.

Cyril (MG): Well, we've not really got a society here. It's everybody for themselves. There is a lot of aggravation and violence. Family life is not like it used to be.

Arthur (MG): You daresn't leave your front door open. You're frightened of getting mugged in the house, let alone going out.

It is violence that emerges as people's major concern with the way society is perceived to be changing. Often this violence is viewed as being perpetrated by the young against their elders. 'Youths' and 'hooligans' seem to have little respect for older people. The reasons for the young turning to violence are varied:

Mary (DW): When you see all these kids and it just disheartens you... They've no respect for themselves, so how can they have respect for anyone else?

Anne (DW): I can't understand it - the young 'uns beating up old people... Bring hanging back, whip for kids and stuff like that. I agree with corporal punishment. Society would be a lot better... People are too namby-pamby with the kids. There's not enough 'clattering' [beating] to me... I don't think children respect their elders at all... It's all right saying 'blame it on unemployment', but people that've been brought up properly shouldn't go and beat old people up or kill or rape someone. To me, it's what society's made them. It's sommat about bringing up. It started in school, and parents have changed.

Michelle (MG): It worries you sick, doesn't it? We were brought up to respect people. There's no respect these days in anybody... It's mainly the teenage bracket. I mean, there is no respect at school for a start. When they get to fourth years, they've no respect for the teachers.

Stuart (MG): It's the trend in general, the general attitude of people, not just children, it's the parents as well because I know for a fact that parents don't care what their children are doing... They've no respect for property, people or anything the youngsters of today.

Doreen (PH): Terrible, the youngsters... Once upon a time, I could only have a ha'penny a week, but now look at what they get now. They buy these glues and go and steal, don't they? Drugs and all that.

Sheila (PH): All the hooligans! You're frightened to go out late at night now. These youngsters, they only seem to be out to see what they can damage. You get them everywhere... Children haven't got anything to do. There's all this unemployment - no jobs.

Linked to crime and violence by many is the issue of unemployment. In this case, violence is not age-related, but the obvious outcome of recent economic changes which have forced more and more people out of paid employment. For many, crime and violence may stem from unemployment:

Albert (DW): Violence is caused, I think, 'cause they've got no work. Half the lads, they've no jobs and haven't had work since they left school... That causes a lot of disagreement. If they've jobs and money, they're all right... If they keep being out of work then or twenty years, well, only way they can get money is to rob people.

Joe (AC): If you send your child to school and in the end there's no job, you got to go on the dole, you begin to wonder what it's all about. Things like this cause the trouble between the youths and the police - it's their bitterness and frustration that they're being treated that way.

Delores (AC): I would like to see all my children, all five of them at work... But Carlton, there's nothing out there for him... and being at home, it makes him angry, and anger it leads to violence.

Miriam (MG): The young ones, I always put that down to them not being able to get jobs, and as far as lads are concerned I think they should have kept the national service on. I don't think so many people would've been taking drugs... It learns them to look after themselves, it learns them to respect people which I think they lack today.

Gareth (PH): As far as crime is concerned, it is terrible. Mugging old people and things like that. Unemployment it has changed a lot.

Unemployment and the associated poverty are viewed as separate and important dimensions of the way British society is changing. The rapid increases in unemployment and poverty in early 1980s are seen to impinge directly on people's senses of well-being and hopes for the future:

Charles (PH): I often wonder what is going to happen when [my children] leave school because there are going to be no jobs for them. The oldest is nine, but as far as I'm concerned, he' got no chance.

Peter (MG): There's a load of lads who are out of work - experienced blokes too. Some of them have got no chance.

Ian (MG): It's all these YTS, cheap labour. Twelve months, then out and somebody else in... It's cheap labour and they don't pay at all, do they? And they get all the menial jobs.

Dennis (DW): I remember one time you could finish a job and straight into another. There's no way now. No way. I've been out of work nearly five years. I've never had a chance of a job. You go down there - money they give you from Social Security ain't enough to live on... When you go for a job, there's 60 or so there - you've got no chance. Even when they leave school nowadays, they've got no chance.

People of pensionable age and the unemployed are particularly at risk from the effects of poverty:

Brenda (PH): A lot of people need heating in their homes. Perhaps a bit more money to heat their.places. If people can afford to eat well and live quite well, that's about as much as you can do... Welfare, I think there could be more done.

Alec (PH): I think the majority of illnesses that are caused with people over 50 is caused by these old places not being adequately warm enough in the winter.

Rita (DW): The heating I have to cut down on because I can't afford it... If it goes cold during the day, I can't do nowt about it. Now me hot water, I have to cut it off completely... Though I need it, I can't have it, I can't afford it. I have to put me kettle on. It's not fair when you've worked all your life.

Nina (DW): I think Maggie [Thatcher] is trying to kill the old 'uns off one by one because with these prices going up the only thing you can save on is coal... Upstairs is terribly cold, but we can't afford to put fires on because of the bills.

Nina brings into focus the ultimate cause, for some, of the unemployment or poverty they suffer. Government policy is often seen as emanating from the Prime Minister and her policies are part of the way in which life in contemporary Britain is becoming more of a struggle and much less pleasant:

> Doreen (PH): Unemployment, strikes. I think it's terrible. The unions are too powerful and the unemployment! At first, she said she was going to help the little man, Margaret Thatcher, but she's shutting down these small places.

> Shobha (AS): The things are very expensive. [The government] is not doing much for us, not for anybody. Look how the young generation are growing up, walking the streets, and they don't get good money from the Social Security. They are jobless and they are robbing houses. We don't like the government, they aren't doing any good for us.

> Delores (AC): Mrs. Thatcher is strong and she is outrageous. She is only one person - why she getting away with it? There's thousands out of work.

> Ivy (AC): I just muddle along with Mrs. Thatcher's ways, waiting for the next election. I go along with everything 'cause there is nothing you can do.

> Pat (DW): I don't think I'd have another baby. I don't think I'd bring another child into the world now. I've very strong political views... I'm very much for nuclear disarmament... Young people of today don't know anything about war, what it means to people, what it's done to people. It's all hushed up.

> Maureen (DW): I'm real militant, me. I think everybody should just down tools and show the sod [Thatcher]. I mean, she couldn't do it if you stood up to it. But she's gonna make it so you can't have a union... Look at Poland. They say it's a wonderful thing, is Solidarity, but in England, it's a joke. While they're over there, it's lovely - here, phoo - rubbish!

For the black respondents, there is the added fear of the Thatcher government tightening further immigration legislation and introducing some form of repatriation:

> Syeda (AS): It is not good. [The government] are making the laws very strict, especially if we have to bring some relatives from Pakistan, or some boy or girl to get married.

> Ruby (AC): They should never have put Mrs. Thatcher there. She talk that she will stop the immigration now, send the blacks back to where they came from. But she can't do it. Mrs. Thatcher no send me home. No deport me.

The National Health Service is also seen to be under threat from the Thatcher policies:

Frank (PH): I could get political and bring Mrs. Thatcher in. I don't like what she's dong to the NHS. At 'Southfields' hospital, the cleaners have been on strike for a year now and it's going to happen elsewhere.

Jim (DW): Them that's got jobs are the lucky ones, so it's up to them. They should pay for [the NHS]. It comes back to government... They cut down on all the important things.

Alec (PH): This national health I don't go much on. When it first came into operation, it was a good thing, but this day and age, this government is proceeding towards private hospitals... Everything she said, she's gone against. I don't think there'll be a national health in a few months' time.

Ivy (AC): Improvements? What a chance when Maggie Thatcher's cutting down on the health service so you're not even sure of getting the right treatment these days.

In their discussions about the way society is changing and what is happening around them, people voice their fears forcefully, but at the same time, they imply a certain degree of pessimism and resignation. As with their health and the likelihood of the incidence of illness, there is a tendency to feel concerned about what is happening, but also to accept the changes and acquiesce with their lot:

Emily (AC): I have no power to change anything. How can I change anything? We can just put in a complaint and see how far it goes that is all.

Wendy (MG): Well, sometimes you think when you listen. But it's happening. Things will happen and that's it. You can't stop it.

Beatrice (DW): News is bad. I don't like to watch it... I keep myself occupied.

Mark (MG): I'm just one of those people who thinks about my mother and myself and that's it. I disagree with vandalism, that's all.

Jean (AC): You cannot change anything.

Deidre (DW): I just accept the way it happens.

Elaine (MG): I don't have time to worry about the outside world.

The 'outside world' is, for most, a depressing and largely unalterable experience. The depressing nature of life in Britain today is further heightened for some by remembering a past in Britain or elsewhere as a better time and/or place. This past may be a Caribbean island, or a close community bathed in imperial grandeur, or a village in rural England or the Indian sub-continent. In making sense of life in Britain, largely by resigning themselves to a rather demoralised state, people have recourse to their historic memory (see chapter 2), a group's conception of the past which is not necessarily consciously regarded as such by that group. Thus for example, Britain's imperial past may engender racist explanations to make sense of the world; or the past in warmer climes may help to mask, nostalgically, the unpleasantness of life in Britain. These images of the past may not be truly representative (in historical terms) of how things were, but they seem real in people's minds and their feelings and actions are rooted in them. Challenges to these 'ideal states' will be resisted as they are pivotal to people's sense of who they are and how they can get through everyday life.

CONCLUSIONS

Living in Britain is the context of people's lives; it is the shared world made up of the personal worlds they live in and experience daily as well as 'external' forces. This context consists of work, racism, locality (see also chapter 3), crime, youth, employment, poverty, violence and Thatcherism. These dimensions determine the nature of British society (see chapter 1) and social change as well as people's perceptions of them. They are mostly unpleasant things, facts of life over which people seem to have little choice. In this, we are not implying that people have no control over their own lives or that there are certain aspects of life over which some people have control and others over which they do not. Societal influences affect all our actions and perceptions, but we only notice these influences through our own perceptions and actions.

The world is there, but it still has to be made sense of. In making sense of it, we use our perceptions and experiences of reality. The world is not, of course, a merely individualistic social construction. Each individual is placed in the world by the forces of work and society in general, and also places her/himself in it through choices between options. There are, then, two interrelated and irreducible worlds: one of personal life in which the individual appears to have some choices and control, and one of societal life in which that choice and control seem constrained. These worlds are not separate entities, but act in relation to each other, as manifested in everyday life. At one time and in some circumstances (such as having a well-paid job), the personal world, in which negotiated meanings and social constructions seems to dominate, may dictate life. At another time, and with different circumstances (such as being out of work) the societal world becomes paramount, with everyday life being constrained by poverty or feelings of poor social worth.

At times, individuals may respond to the world by acquiescing or being demoralised; at others by criticising. These responses can be seen clearly in people's views about living in Britain in this chapter. The basis of their criticism lies in the personal world in which perceptions and experiences combine to challenge this other-world rationality with another. They can criticise, and many do, but their criticism is often muted by the realisation that they can do little to change the way things are. By criticising, they can gain some power over what is happening, but they know this control is illusory. Most, then, feel they must accept things as they are, but social change in Britain today has few positive features. For most, their quality of life is being reduced by factors such as unemployment, racism, violence. In this context, health becomes one (significant) aspect of life in general, part, as this chapter has averred, of well-being and quality of life. Edith summarises the relationship:

> Edith (DW): If you've no money, you can't do a lot of things. Finance and your health - if you've got those, you can ride mountains, can't you? If you've no money and bad health, you've all the problems in the world. And one brings on the other.

Life in Britain is the context of health, yet health is an integral element of living in Britain. They are dialectically related, just as are the personal and societal worlds. The interrelations of these worlds can be seen in a specific realm of health, in the ways that people cope with illnesses.

5 'You have to use your loaf': coping with illness

We are not specifically interested in how people cope psychologically, socially or economically with specific bouts or types of illness. We are rather concerned with how they deal in general terms, with, and manage, ill-health, i.e. with the strategies which are adopted when people see themselves on these and related issues, e.g. how people know that they are ill, how they perceive their symptoms, how they use health care facilities. Social scientists treat these strategies as 'illness behaviour.'(1) As we shall see, a common strategy for coping is ignoring the problem and it is estimated that some 75 to 80 per cent of all symptoms are managed and/or treated without referral to doctors.(2) (We examine formal care in the next chapter.) And many of the symptoms presented to doctors are discussed by the ill person with other lay people before attending the surgery.(3) While coping and its associated referral and consultation patterns are complex, individuals are likely to consult with spouse, parents (usually the mother), friends and relatives in dealing with a bout of ill-health.(4) It may be that social networks of advice-giving and coping strategies exist which individuals may utilise.(5) Family and kin and friends are used differently(6) and may in fact provide different kinds of help, with kin assistance implying long term commitments, permanent ties and much give-and-take, and friendship networks supplying knowledge of professionals outside the primary group.(7) Although they seem intuitively important for coping, social networks have seldom been examined the same way in the different studies. In our discussion we shall, therefore, not explicitly concentrate on networks but on the forms which coping strategies take amongst our respondents.

IGNORING, WAIT-AND-SEE, AND TAKING CARE

Coping with illness takes many forms, and can encompass several different attempts to deal with one particular condition. One of the simplest and easiest forms of coping is to ignore the illness. This is often the first reaction to the perception of something wrong with the body, and as we have seen in chapter 2, some people with severe and/or long standing complaints also manage to ignore them in order to consider themselves 'healthy'. The pressures of everyday life on these and others are often such that this way of coping is seen to be the only viable possibility, especially when evidence of the condition can be hidden from others. This disregarding of illnesses can itself take several forms. Some individuals simply dismiss a complaint and carry on with normal life, hoping that it will go away. Indeed 'normal' life is the key to understanding this strategy:

Joyce (PH): I don't let it get me down. I just carry on as normal.

Nick (DW): If you fight [illness], you've got a chance it won't come back again... Tell yourself you haven't got it and try to work it off.

Steve (MG): I just keep going on, I don't worry about it too much.

Sufiya (AS): I don't want to bother for small things. I just leave it and think and hope it will go away on its own.

Some, like Sufiya, are willing to rest or wait until their own bodily resistance will get rid of their symptoms. It is again a form of ignoring, manifested as a 'wait and see' approach:

Gordon (PH): Backache... While it's painful, you don't feel like doing anything. You have to use your loaf and not do anything when it's painful.

Earl (AC): Most of the common things you get disappear within two or three days, so with or without medicine doesn't make any difference.

Paul (AC): I always believe that if you get an illness, your natural body resistance will get rid of it.

A common reaction to a recognised symptom or a chronic condition is to alter one's lifestyle so as not to cause undue pain or difficulty. In this way, long-term conditions can be ignored because they no longer impinge on daily life:

Matt (PH): I did have a disc crushed [in my back]... As soon as I put weight on, it starts affecting me. If I keep my weight down, its O.K.

Ivy (AC): I take precautions [with my health] fearing in

case my hypertension might rise again. I take it easy,
not rushing about.

Beatrice (DW): It's my knees... Osteoarthritis. It's
'cause I'm getting old, me bones are crumbling... I can't
kneel. Mind you, I've no need to kneel - I've got a
vacuum and a mop.

Maud (DW): It's restrictive movement. I can't bend down
very well. I don't wear such things as laced shoes if I
can avoid it... I've sort of got myself into a routine
now that when I have done so much, like a bit of cleaning
up and that, if I feel [the back pain] coming on, well,
that's it, I down tools and sort of rest it while it goes
off.

Eleanor (MG): Well, I couldn't join the police force!...
I don't jog, but I don't want to. I've got a bike, I can
ride that.

Often more than one type of coping strategy is used, in a sort
of chain. Firstly, it may be ignored and 'worked' through;
then some activities may be suspended as it is hoped the
symptoms will disappear; then some action may be taken:

Pat (DW): I get pre-menstrual tension, so I just have to
try to relax all the time... If everything gets on top
of me now, I make sure all the kids are safe and nothing
can happen and then dash upstairs and lay on the bed for
ten minutes and get myself back down.

Leroy (AC): [When I get ill] I just carry on. Unless it
gets worse, then I go to the doctor.

Mary (DW): There's lots of things I can't do [because of
the arthritis], but on the whole I try to keep going, keep
the joints going. It's mainly the spine, arms and hands -
gripping, taking curtains down, anything that is above.

This strategy of ignoring or discounting symptoms or altering
one's life around an illness, is, of course, a form of
psychological coping. Conditions are thought to be
unimportant or are forced away:

Joe (AC): It's a matter of mind over matters.

SMOKING

Some people rely on something to help them cope with
illnesses. They need a 'crutch' to help them overcome
problems (including symptoms) which arise in everyday life.
Joe's use of the strength of his mind is akin to others using
religion or smoking to offset particular concerns and
especially 'worry' or 'stress'. We have already seen in
chapter 3 that smoking is viewed ambivalently. The health
education and medical messages that it is detrimental to

health are not easily accepted when many feel that smoking has soothing, calming effects which help to counterbalance worries which are perceived to cause very serious conditions. Some may use this argument as an excuse for smoking to which they are addicted, but the use of smoking for some is clearly important for alleviating stress and even chesty coughs!

> Paul (DW): I think I'm too old to worry now. I've tried to stop smoking a few times, but as I say I get depressed as it is and when I try to stop smoking, I lead (my wife) a dog's life. It's more or less just to calm my nerves down.

> Frances (DW): It does your nerves good. If you're suffering with your nerves, it calms you down... I stopped before until my husband had his heart attack and that with nerves put me on again.

> Doris (MG): It does [help] if you've got a cough... you can get it off your chest easier... It does help your nerves.

> Janet (PH): [Smoking] helps with your breathing and that because I get chesty.

> Audrey (PH): You could walk across the road and get run over... It helps me, it helps my nerves.

> Marian (PH): I did give it up, but then I separated from my husband and found it was better to have a cigarette than a drink, so I had one.

For some of the women, it is likely that if they go to their general practitioner for their 'nerves' or depression, they will be offered tranquilizers of some sort. Some of these women (men do not seem to be prescribed tranquilizers routinely for depressive disorders) prefer to cope by smoking rather than with tablets:

> Pat (DW): Smoking is bad for your health, but I still do it... It does worry me, but it does help me... I'd rather smoke five-a-day than be hooked on tranquilizers all my life.

Some of the respondents of Afro-Caribbean descent mention using marijuana to cope by reducing stress:

> Earl (AC): I smoke cigarettes or hash or marijuana from time to time... It helps you, thought wise, I think. It seems to open up your mind, relax you.

RELIGION

For others, particularly the Asian women and older women of Afro-Caribbean descent, it is religion rather than smoking that helps them to cope with the pressures of everyday life. Religious beliefs are a source of solace and strength, and so soothe away worries in a similar way to smoking, but they also have far-reaching effects on individuals' ways of life. Not only does religion affect a person's state of mind, but it also provides rules that affect life-style. In short, it provides a moral map of the world. Illness has a particular place in this scheme. For some, illnesses are seen as punishment for wrong deeds, but on the whole religious beliefs seem to project the inevitability of illness and provide ways of coping and recovering through God or faith in God:

Delores (AC): I'm not afraid of getting nothing. Whatever coming to me, you got to take it. What's the point of being afraid? Whatever is coming will come to you, so what good is worrying? Whatever it is, you have to carry it and look to the bible or whatever to help you through it.

Ivy (AC): My great enjoyment is going to church... I can go into church for half and hour, and then when I go home, I feel quite refreshed, peaceful, and I forget all the aggro at work and I think about the scripture and the powers.

Louise (AC): I never cry, just call on Him, because He is there to help me in all my needs. I have faith in God. I don't take tablets. God is always there with me, to heal... When I go for the op., God always revives me quick.

Naseem (AS): Prayer helps very much, even when you are very depressed. It would help more than the tranquilizers... Those who believe in God and pray to God, they must be certainly healthier than the others, mentally and physically.

Tanseem (AS): You are more peaceful when you are praying to God and more relaxed. It eases the worries.

Sufiya (AS): Religion helps a lot. When my child was ill, my mother-in-law prayed a lot and we gave charity to the poor and sometimes I think that may be my child is getting better due to the prayers rather than the medicine.

Geeta (AS): Prayers are more helpful than the medicine.

Frank (PH): The medics will tell you it is impossible to come off that many [12 barbiturates a day] - 10 is enough to kill someone who is not used to them!... It was O.K. just peace in Christ.

Lilian (PH): You should be able to talk to Him all the time. It doesn't matter where you are... If you've got problems, you should talk to Him about it. He is the Great Psychiatrist.

Religion, then, like smoking, acts mainly as a coping

strategy by releasing tension and thus avoiding undue worry, which as we saw in chapter 3 was isolated as one of the major causes of ill-health. Religion and smoking are forms of mental coping. They provide relief (smoking) and strength (religion), but they also give people the ability to discard or discount symptoms. Religion, for example, gives the older woman of Afro-Caribbean descent strength to cope with pressures but it also enables them to disregard prejudice and discrimination. Smoking has advantages and disadvantages: it relieves stress and gives some pleasure, but it may also be a contributary cause of cancer or heart disease. In weighing up both sides, some feel unable to accept smoking and/or religious faith as coping strategies. There are, however, other ways of coping which involve more physical applications. Many involve 'medicine' - a concept which may include such things as home remedies, particular foods or drinks, proprietary drugs and 'alternative' methods of health care.

EXERCISE AND DIET

We have already seen that some believe that lack of exercise may be regarded as a cause of ill-health (Chapter 3). Exercise is a way of ensuring well-being, and is a form of coping through being preventative, as is diet. Some feel they get enough exercise at work or through ordinary daily activities:

> Joe (AC): I work very hard. I do a lot of walking - must be 4 or 5 miles a shift... When the eight hours finish, I get enough exercise and I'm all worn out.

> Rani (AS): I do exercise enough because of our prayer. You have to exercise, bending down, standing up, bowing. Five times a day - that is enough!

> Des (DW): My work's exercise for me.

> Stuart (MG): I do a lot of exercise at work - walking and lifting.

Exercise helps to keep the body 'in good shape' and thus able to fend off some illnesses:

> Syeda (AS): [Exercise] is very good. You stay smart and active and your body stays in order.

> Leroy (AC): It's very important to keep your body in good shape... If you look after your body, I think, in the long run, you'll be better off than someone who don't.

As we outlined in chapter 3, most people accept that diet may have important effects on their health, but seldom feel able or inclined to do much about it. There is, however, an obvious concern expressed about the types and quality of food they are able to buy and its possible effects on health. This concern has been mirrored in (or perhaps initiated by) media coverage of food and it constituents. There are particular worries about additives:

> Kevin (PH): All the additives and things they are putting in the food now... We have started to watch what we eat.

> Jack (DW): They put that much stuff in now, don't they? Chemicals in food these days. You don't know what you're eating half the time.

> Earl (AC): It must be something to do with all these additives they put in food and things they feed to the cows to produce more milk; chickens to produce different colour eggs... There's got to be an answer for that, because years ago, you didn't hear of cancer.

Not only are foods seen to be increasingly full of additives, but they are processed or frozen so that they last longer. These processes are thought to diminish the goodness of the food, thus reducing the preventative powers of a good diet:

> Gordon (PH): There's foods like fatty foods that are detrimental - well, can bring on stomach complaints which would lead to something else. Food is important - you've got to be careful with it... Vegetables, of course, today they aren't much good. By the time you've got them half frozen to your table, they don't look very appetizing.

> Tim (PH): The food we eat now is totally 100% rubbish. Everything. Years ago, after the war, foods changed because of the conditions. Now it is terrible - they spray all the crops and everything. Most of the stuff is frozen, processed, tinned. I think the food is terrible today.

> Delores (AC): We eat too much ice. The meat, it take away all the [variety and strength]. We eat that, That is trash... All the nourishment has gone into the ice.

> Ruby (AC): Since I came here and you eat and you don't have no health for the food is not fresh... We have to get the frozen meat and heat it and that's why we don't have our health.

> Louise (AC): The food here is fridged, frozen. It is not fresh. All this food is no good. We're eating it - all right, it won't kill us, but the fresh food is best.

> Indira (AS): The meat in this country is not fresh and frozen meat is not very good for health. In our country [India] you go straight to the butcher and get fresh meat, but in this county, the meat is very stale.

As is mentioned explicitly above, the food of today does not compare favourably with the food remembered in the past:

> Mary (DW): None of the foods have got proper stuff in,

have they? The vegetables have all got fertilizer on. It's not like it were in olden days when it were just manure and goodness in the soil.

Anne (DW): They say they're healthy foods we're eating. Me, we used to go to school and have dinners - a set dinner, and we used to eat it and puddings after it. And to me, nowadays when they go down to school dinners, they get beefburgers and stuff like that. I think it's them main foods and fresh foods we used to get that build up your resistance. Now there's all sorts [of viruses] going round. Kids always seem to be off school with summat or other... When we were young, there were no fridges. We used to the fresh food and there were nowt of this stuff they are spraying. To me, I seemed an healthier kid than what my kids are.

Miriam (MG): Food isn't like it used to be. They force it and chickens are battery fed. I think that when they were free range and the animals went out and was grazing, I think the food was much better, tasted much better... I think they have put too many colourings and too many things in.

With all the different sources of advice about what constitutes a 'healthy' diet, it is not surprising that there are many views about what people 'should' eat. Some rely on their own experience; others on special diets. Many mentioned that variety is important, or the balancing of different types of food:

Gerald (PH): I like to eat plenty of fibre and very little fat. It's not so much the calories I'm interested in as the balance between carbohydrate and protein.

Winnie (DW): We just have stews and things like that we think are good. Summer salads, fresh fruit, that kind of thing.

Earl (AC): A balance of vegetables. The meats, they're not so important, but it's the vitamins, proteins, natural fibres.

Martha (AC): If you can balance your food it's all right. Bit of this, bit of that, plenty of greens and just balance the starches... If you always stick to a balanced diet, I think your health will be all right.

Other emphasise particular foods or cooking methods which help to maintain a healthy diet and hence a healthy life:

Alec (PH): When you start doing away with, or save a few shillings on food, that's when you start to deteriorate. I've always been used to three meals a day. I look after myself.

Vera (DW): I always make myself a good meal. I don't let

my food go.

Beatrice (DW): I like my dinner and then I have owt for my tea, but I always have a good dinner every day.

Carlton (AC): Tradition - West Indian food, I take it as the strongest part of my living.

To eat a 'proper' diet, then, is considered essential. It is not only for the maintenance of good health, but also that an individual can be seen to be looking after her or himself, not encouraging neglect and so doing as much as anyone can to prevent the onset of illness.

It is interesting in many of the quotations about food to notice the presence of a concern with a healthier diet, as promoted by the Health Education Authority, British Medical Association and various government exhortations. Several people mention that they are trying to change their diets away from sweet and fried foods towards more fibre and less fat:

Doreen (PH): Oh yes, I do believe in this high fibre business and vegetable fats rather than animal fat.

Frank (PH): I've tried to alter my diet because I think that is important. I avoid white sugar and salt and stuff and I think that helps [against the pains in my hands]... I also use garlic and I'm a person that never gets colds... I chew on a clove of garlic. Doesn't make me popular, like, but I don't give in.

Jean (AC): It depends on what food you're going to eat. If you're going to stuff yourself with fatty foods and sweet things, you might as well not bother.

Enda (DW): We used to have fried stuff, but it's all grilled now and my dad says eat fresh fruit and vegetables.

Julie (DW): Instead of eating potatoes, I have more vegetables - peas and cabbage. On a Saturday morning, when (the family) is having a fried breakfast, I'll have two boiled eggs. They have butter; I have slimming margarine.

Although some people are, undoubtedly, moving towards the prescribed 'healthy diet', it is also the case that most of the people in this study are not. Expert pronouncements about foods and diets do not always accord with people's own views on the merits of their traditional diets. There are also those who agree superficially that a high fibre diet may be good for their health, but who have not adopted any of its foods. A few discuss the importance of food for health altogether:

Betty (MG): I ask my son what he wants, and if he wants beans on toast, he'll have beans on toast, egg or sausage.

To tell you the truth, I don't think we look bad on what we've eaten. To me, I can eat anything.

Joan (MG): You can get your health just from eating ordinary food.

'Health foods' are dismissed by many as 'fads' 'gimmics' or because they have been tried but are seen to be expensive and/or unappetising:

Tony (PH): We ventured into one or two things, but here doesn't seem to be too much taste to me... and they're expensive.

Len (MG): I think there are things on the normal market that you can buy without paying for the expensive health foods.

Andy (DW): Crap, innit? Definitely.

Edith (DW): I don't think they're necessary if you're having a proper diet. If you have a proper diet, all them pills and vitamins and health foods, you don't need them.

Mona (DW): I went onto one of those bran fibre diets and had a lot of trouble with my stomach... They found it was the bran that was doing it and it blows you up... I find that beans seem to give me this wind, so I have cut all things like this out.

Maud (DW): I think a lot of these [health foods] are gimmics.

The 'official' (HEA, BMA, government) idea of a healthy diet corresponds quite closely with the traditional diet of those of Asian descent. Despite this, there have been campaigns funded by the government to fight rickets which have directly attacked Asian diets because they are said to be low in Vitamin D. Asian diets are criticised because they do not contain oily fish such as mackerel and because many choose to eat butter rather than artificially fortified margarine.(8) Advice to Asians to eat margarine rather than butter does not accord with the views about the purity and health-giving nature of butter and other dairy produce:

Reena (AS): We use pure ghee [clarified butter], milk and butter to keep us healthy... Butter is good for health - it gives energy.

Tanseem (AS): Because we were farmers, we had fresh milk, pure butter and vegetables... This kind of things we used to keep in our house to keep us healthy.

Indira (AS): We never used medicine, but we took lots of pure milk, butter and yogurt. Because we had cows in our home, we could have all these things fresh.

Another traditional theory held by those of Asian descent which is challenged by western views concerns weight. Several of the women express the view that to be fat is healthy, an idea which may well have developed because malnutrition is an obvious sign of poverty. They show their concern particularly when discussing their children:

Naseem (AS): One [of my sons] is very healthy, very tall and he eats very well. The other son is small and he doesn't eat very much at all and I am worried about him.

Dalee (AS): The eldest child is healthier than the other -the small one is a bit slim... but now the little one is also getting fat, so I am happy.

As indicated in chapter 2, the Asian respondents also have a theory about balancing hot and cold forces in the body. Some illnesses are seen to be brought about by an imbalance between hot and cold. To redress this balance, and, one hopes, to restore health, hot or cold foods and drinks can be taken, depending on the condition. This is another way, then, in which the diet can act as a coping strategy:

Rani (AS): You have to get a balance in the bile of the body - the hot things cause you bile and heat in the body and then it upsets your stomach... so to balance them you have to take some cold things.

Naseem (AS): [Measles is] a very hot disease. It can make the children very ill, the temperature is very high... They can't eat chicken, meat, eggs, and so on because they are very hot foods... They used to think that egg, chicken, dried fruit, are very hot, so you shouldn't eat very much of them because they will raise your blood pressure or make you bleed too much... There are certain foods that they think are cold, like fruit, vegetables, carrots etc., and these are good for your health... cold things, they are good for your health, and hot food is not very good.

Tasneem (AS): Certain spices which we think are hot, they can upset your stomach and they upset your head... They used to say that oranges were very cold, so don't eat oranges in cold weather, they will give you headache.

There is a disjuncture in some cases between traditional and Western/modern ideas about diet and health. Traditional beliefs are, of course, not irrational, but are simply ordered in different ways and for different purposes, having developed under very different circumstances. They may in a rational way contradict Western ideas and this contradiction may lead to individuals questioning both their traditional theories and Western ones, sometimes trying to hold two competing views of health and diet:

Nassem (AS): They think in this country that slim people

are healthier than fat people, but I don't know, sometimes the slim people are also ill... In our community, they think fat people are healthier, but fat people are more liable to certain illnesses like blood pressure, heart disease... I don't know.

Tasneem (AS): You can never really tell who is a really healthy person. Some fat people are healthy, some are ill. Some people who are thin are very healthy. Some people are slim due to the illness.

Shobha (AS): Average weight people are healthier than the fat. The fat people have some problems - so do the thin.

These competing views are also expressed by some whites:

Sandra (DW): Nowadays they say 'meat and potato pie ain't good for you, red meat ain't good for you.' All things like that. But I mean, we were brought up on that...

Mick (DW): I don't think they ever worried about their diet because they had to concern themselves with what they could get...

Sandra (DW): I think a lot of animal fat ain't good for you, and a lot of fried stuff - fish and chips. But they used to tell us fish and chips were the most nutritious food you could eat... I am a big believer in milk and now they say milk is not good for you...

Mick (DW): Well, you see, we are confused, utterly confused... Basic food is best. If they stopped getting technical with it, it would be a lot better.

SELF-MEDICATION AND HOME REMEDIES

Food can be used in a preventative way, by building on the body's natural defences, but it is also the basis of self-medication. Food, although not a medicine in the strict sense, is a major source of this self-medication, and others include proprietary drugs, herbal and home remedies, and tonics. Advice on the particular remedy to adopt for an illness is often sought from family and/or friends, and the largest bank of knowledge is held by the older women. The remedies are, then, literally 'old wives tales', often with their roots in traditional culture. They can be found among all the groups of respondents but it is those of Afro-Caribbean descent who mention and use the most. They use some remedies regularly, and almost always try something before thinking of consulting their G.P. If an illness is recognised, the appropriate remedy will be tried for about three days before further help is sought.

Specific preparations are used for particular illnesses. For colds, for example, several things are recommended:

'Camphorated oil to rub on the chest and glands' and 'ferrol compounds' (Ivy); 'black coffee and a squeeze of lemon' (Delores) - with the addition of, 'a strong drink, like Bacardi' (Leroy); 'ferrol tonic' (Delores); 'Honey and lemon' (Judy); 'peppermint tea, or spice or ginger tea' (Louise, Jean and Joe); and 'bayrum' (Danny).

Joe and Jean have an exceptionally large range of home remedies, although Joe admits that, "You can't get them very easy here. Some of the time you can get them from health shops", or from a local 'druggist'. He speaks of fever grass, 'black mint', ginger and lime, to be made into teas to make you "sweat it out and be better in no time"; 'wintergreen', 'sloe linament' and 'Canadian stuff' for bites and wasp stings; 'bisodol' or 'hunters' for his ulcer; and 'bitter hollows' for biliousness. Some of these preparations are produced under brand-names.

Ivy speaks of 'bayrum', a poultice made of bay leaves, and a popular Jamaican remedy for headaches and feverish feelings; as well as cod-liver oil, 'for the bowel system.' Martha recommends 'cleansing herbs', "for bowels and it regulate the blood... and cure like what we call rheumatism pains." Delores recommends 'cod liver malt', which "clear out your bowels and keeps your system working", and she adds, tastes better than cod liver oil. She also speaks of bayrum, grated onion and sugar for whooping cough, and she tells how a nutmeg put in her father's cheek helped him to regain feeling and movement after a stroke. Herbal teas are ubiquitous, being used by all the informants in all the islands represented: Barbados, Jamaica and Dominica.

Specific aspects of the workings of the body, particularly the blood and bowel systems, are the targets for many of the remedies. It can be seen that most of the recipes cause sweating, or 'clean out the bowels', or regulate the blood. Delores and Joe have well-worked out theories about the blood. Delores says (this being echoed by Martha), "The older you get, your blood gets thinner and you get weaker", and so,by implication, one needs tonics. Joe's theory is quite different from this: "the blood in the body is thicker here than in the Tropics... I think that cause a lot of this heart disease" (Joe). His theory originates from his mechanical knowledge that, "If you put water through a pump, it will sent it through quick", whereas, "with oil, it's much slower... I just draw my own conclusion that if the blood was to run thinner, it wouldn't put a strain on the heart" (Joe).

Tonics are also mentioned. These are used to 'wash out' the bowels, to relax (e.g. marijuana or ganga, smoked or used as a tea or mixed with rum), or to build the body up. Proprietary brands such as 'Wincarnis' and 'Sanatogen' are used, as well as 'Strongback' made from sea-weed. Two of the young men have devised tonics of their own, consisting of eggs, milk, sugar, Guinness and carrot juice (Leroy and Earl). Alcholic spirits can also be taken as tonics, as well as to relieve colds.

This obvious wealth of remedies amongst the respondents of Afro-Caribbean descent does not seem to be repeated amongst the other groups. Only a few of those of Asian descent mentioned using herbs (Reena and Rajinda) or spices such as ginger or garlic (Rajinda and Tasneem) as specific remedies. Few were willing to admit having seen a hakim, a traditional practitioner, who sells herbal treatments, because, they said, the hakims treat mainly the poorest people who cannot afford Western doctors. Some of the white respondents mentioned home remedies:

Miriam (MG): I think [home remedies] are better for you, as well. I don't believe in taking all those tablets they give you. You know, if I go to the doctor's and he gives me tablets, I've got to be truthful, I might take one or two and as soon as I feel better,that's it, throw them away.

Stuart (MG): Backaches - I remember my mum and dad and my grandmother using Sloe's linament which used to do the trick. Half the tables we get do nothing... I've stopped going to [the doctor] with backaches - I just get Disprin.

Paul (DW): My eldest daughter, she's mentally handicapped... and she gets bedsores... A nurse had an old remedy of putting honey on the sores and it's a long time since she's had any sores now.

Pat (DW): Get a fresh swede, chop it up with a tablespoon of brown sugar and leave it overnight in the fridge and the syrup that comes off it is absolutely marvellous... It makes like a cough linctus.

Winnie (DW): Mixing honey, glycerine and lemon to loosen a cough... We find it as good as anything.

CHEMISTS, FAITH HEALERS AND 'ALTERNATIVE' PRACTITIONERS

Whites also rely more than the others on local pharmacists who may be asked for, or offer, advice:

Alison (DW): My husband has psoriasis and he pays for his own ointment from the chemist... We know Clive at the chemist's so we ask him if he can recommend anything.

Anthony (DE): I get transvestin [ointment] from the chemist. I use it regular for aches and pains... And vitamin tablets, all sorts - alfalfa, brewer's yeast, vitamin C, E, B complex, wheat-germ, sunflower seeds.

Phyllis (DW): I get linctus at chemist. I dunno what it's called - he just make it up.

Gordon (PH): I'm taking these herbal salts. There's one for chest colds and coughs and this one's for a bit of sinus trouble... These I take in the morning now... They're salts, so they're natural.

Others in Parkheath buy preparations such as indigestion tablets, bar-beans for bowels, cough medicine and linament for muscle injuries. In Mossley Green, they advocate the use of tea with sennapods or brimstone and treacle, vinegar for headaches, hen's fat for coughs, wool dipped in camphorated oil and butter and sugar for sore throats, lemon juice or hot milk and brandy for colds, golden-eye ointment and kaolin poultices for boils. In Deanswood, others mention aludrox for indigestion and lem-sip for colds.

Most of the home remedies and proprietary drugs mentioned above are used on physical illnesses. If the symptoms persist, and ignoring the complaint or trying home remedies or pharmacist's advice fail to have any effects, people may turn to their GPs or to 'alternative' practitioners or methods. Some will use alternative methods at an early stage in the illness, others as a last resort after all has failed. They represent another choice or coping strategy.

Amongst those of Afro-Caribbean descent, there are some who attend fundamentalist churches which practise faith healing. One of the whites has also tried this:

Delores (AC): We see a lot of people come there sick, stroke, can't walk... what we use is olive oil - massage that oil, praying water - we pray and the one who can see, whom God raised to do that, him massage them.

Ruby (AC): If you sick, they pray for you, heal you and you get better. Is only the Almighty God you must put your trust to.

Ray (PH): We believe that the power of Jesus is still present in the world to heal today... I did't think I had a particular gift of healing from God, but I prayed for a deaf lady and she began to hear. I prayed for a lady with kidney disease and her hands were all swollen and the swelling went down.

The others who have used 'alternative' medicine have visited homeopaths, herbalists and osteopaths:

Lilian (PH): I went to see a homeopath... and he said to me, 'you are in deep depression.' Well, if you go round to my doctor's, he doesn't look at your eyes and say, 'You are in deep depression.' A homeopath did, but it cost 20 pounds, just for one. I mean, you just can't afford that. I am on social security.

Claire (PH): Dr. Perkin's he's a psychiatrist and a homeopathic doctor. He spent nearly two hours with me, went through case history, listened, put over his point and I've got a lot more confidence in him... I've been reading over a year about herbal treatments and alternative medicine which I am very interested in and I 'phoned up the Fellowship of Homeopaths in London and asked them to recommend one... 30 pounds for the first consultation with treatment and tablets. I've got to go back in a fortnight and that is 18 pounds consultation and tablets... I'd rather pay that and get the attention and ask questions and not get ushered out than take a tranquilizer... I 'm intelligent. I don't need sedatives. I need help to get to the main problem.

Dalee (AS): The first stroke happened because the lady next door told me I should have homeopathic treatment for the pains, this arthritis... At that time, the doctor had put me on steroids, always I am on steroids. Well, I stopped the steroids to take the homeopathic drug, and then the stroke happened. Now I always take the steroids... My doctor said that if they could find him [the homeopathic doctor] they will sue him. First of all when I had the stroke, he didn't want to know anything at all. Then later, he said, 'Forget about me, and just go to the hospital.' (The first stroke left Dalee paralysed down one side, which makes her virtually house-bound and leaves her unable to do all but the most simple tasks.)

Marian (PH): I had a car accident and the bottom vertebra was broken. It's all right unless I lift something. The doctor and hospital can't help me at all, something they can't find, but an osteopath treats it. I don't like paying for it, but he's good.

CONCLUSIONS

In this chapter we have examined what may be termed 'lay' or 'alternative' methods of coping - in other words, they do not involve the formal medical care system. They are typically used on minor ailments, recognised illnesses or conditions which the doctor/hospital system has been unable to treat successfully. These lay methods are closely related to people's perceptions of illness (Chapter 2) and their theories of causation (Chapter 3). Illnesses caused by 'germs' may need 'sweating out' with the use of strong drinks, or eased by eating (or not eating) particular foods. The old saying 'Feed a cold, starve a fever', has relevance here.

Coping in these terms usually involves taking food or medicine to ease or cure physical complaints. There is also an element of 'mental coping' which is also employed to ease the conditions and difficulties of everyday life. These methods, such as smoking and diets, may contradict accepted Western medical opinion, but they continue to be used because they offer some comfort, satisfaction or enjoyment. Smoking and religious faith in particular can be used by people to gain some control over their daily lives and should be seen as rational responses to circumstances and problems. Smoking and aspects of diet will not be changed just because doctors and governments assert that they are unhealthy. They may be a necessary crutch or traditional practice and, as such, the notion that they may be injurious to health must be ignored, weighed against their psychological advantages.

In most cases, people attempt to control their symptoms and illnesses, without recourse to doctors, at least in the initial stages. Some people do this by ignoring symptoms; others draw on a wealth of experiences and traditional recipes for home remedies. Some use the fringes of the formal medical system, the pharmacists, or attend 'alternative' practitioners. The other form of coping, referral to a G.P. or hospital, is often not a 'higher' form of coping, but last resort. In this case, the individual usually has to give up control over her/his symptoms and body and entrust her/himself to the highly trained medical practitioner. This relaxation of control is not, however, final. Home remedies may continue to be used, and if the doctor's advice does not accord with their perceptions of their needs, they may take back their control, and look elsewhere for help:

> Pat (DW): If it's an illness that's new to me, I usually go straight to the doctor, but once it's been confirmed that it is what I thought it was, usually... I try to deal with it myself... If you don't get satisfaction from your doctor, go to a herbalist!

For the majority, however, an important, if final, point of referral is the formal health care system, to which we now turn.

FOOTNOTES

1. For illness behaviour, see the discussion in R. Dingwall, Aspects of illness, Martin Robertson, 1976; D. Mechanic, Medical sociology, Free Press, 1978.

2. See L. Eisenberg and A. Kleinman (eds). The relevance of social science for medicine, D. Reidel. 1981.

3. Three out of four consult lay people before attending surgery. See E.A. Suchman, Socio-medical variations among ethnic groups, American Journal of Sociology 70, 1964, 319-31.

4. On the lay referral system, see E. Freidson, Profession of dominance, Dodd Mead, 1970, and U. Ignu, Stages in health seeking, Social Science and Medicine 13A, 1979, 445-56. The importance of relatives is discussed by A. Scrambler et al., Kinship and friendship networks and women's demands for primary care, Journal of the Royal College of General Practitioners 26, 746 - 50.

5. See J. McKinlay, Social network influences on morbid episodes and the career of help seeking in L. Eisenberg and A. Kleinman (eds), The relevance of social science for medicine, D. Reidel, 1981.

6. J. Salloway and P. Dillon, A comparison of family networks and friend networks in health care utilisation, Journal of Comparative Family Studies 4, 1973, 131-42.

7. A. Horwitz, Family, kin and friend networks in psychiatric help-seeking, Social Science and Medicine 12, 1978, 297-304.

8. These issues are explored by H. Sheiham and A. Quick, The rickets report, Haringey CHC and CRC, 1982; J. Donovan, Ethnicity and health, Social Science and Medicine 19, 1984, 663-70.

6 'Troubling the doctor': experiences of the formal health-care system

As indicated in chapter five, people cope with illness in a variety of ways, one of which is the consultation of a General Practitioner (GP); another is the attendance at a hospital Accident or Emergency (A&E) Department. Far from being people's first choice of treatment when illness or discomfort is perceived, the formal health care system, except for A & E departments, is often the one of last resort. Some people do go to the GP regularly and often, but the majority are fearful of 'troubling the doctor', usually trying home remedies or over-the-counter drugs first, or just ignoring the problem, hoping it will go away. When people do choose to make appointments or visit their GPs, they have expectations which they hope will be met, based upon their own experiences or those of close friends and/or relatives. When the consultation runs as expected and the outcome is understood and appreciated, the doctor's reputation is enhanced - the 'good' doctor. If, however, the doctor prescribes something that is unwanted or unusual, or behaves in an unexpected manner, the advice and/or prescription may be rejected and the doctor criticised.

In general terms, the majority of people say they are happy with their GPs, and feel that they receive good or adequate treatment. This view may reflect all aspects of health care for those who will never say a bad word about 'their' doctor. There are others, however, who will proffer this view initially, but who will later tell a story in which they severely criticise the same, previously praised, GP. In offering positive opinions about health care, they may be reflecting their subordinate position in the medical arena, acquiescing to medicine's domination and social control. They may also be offering the publicly acceptable view of doctors while privately being much more critical. (Both these issues are discussed in chapter 2). Further, by criticising a dominant system, they may be trying to regain the power and control over their own bodies that they are obliged to devolve to their doctor during the consultation. In short, their criticism may help them to reflect upon what happened and regain the 'upper hand' so that their behaviour and/or problems become beyond approach. Some have had very unpleasant experiences, particularly in hospital but also with GPs.

GENERAL PRACTITIONERS

It is the GP who is the first point of contact with the formal health care system for the majority. Many people want to emphasise that they do not go to their GP without 'good' or 'proper' cause, and that they often go long after the first onset of a problem, or only when it becomes uncontrollable by other means or unbearable:

> Carlton (AC): I like to have a go [with home remedies] and if I can't handle it, I go to the doctor's... I know in some cases doctors are best, but in some cases, I don't need to go to the doctor - like only serious injuries, or something I don't know what's wrong with me... Then I have to go to the doctor. Only time I go.

> Ivy (AC): I delayed going to the doctor about my hypertension because I don't like bothering the doctor. I'd rather use my bayrum.

> Martha (AC): I don't go very often to the doctor. If you're not sick, you just get a common pain in your arm or knee, ankle, you try your own remedy... If it gets worse, you just bear it.

> Peter (MG): It's very rare I have to use them, unless I have to .

> Michelle (MG): I would rather make it up there than call him out. All the years, especially when the kids were babies, I think I've never called the doctor out more than three times. I think they appreciate that.

> Janet (PH): I don't take my children up to the doctor unless they're absolutely bad.

> Alison (DW): I only go to the doctor when I'm forced. Otherwise I don't go. None of us do. Rather than trail to the doctor or even bother with the doctor, we prefer to buy our own stuff from the chemist.

> Pat (DW): There are a lot of things I'd sooner do myself. I'd never go to the doctor with a stupid, trivial complaint like a cold. I'd sooner treat that myself than worry the doctor with it.

> Indira (AS): I don't go because he will just give me the same medicine. It's no use going.

Tanseem (AS): Sometimes I think I should go, but I just leave it.

Bearing these comments in mind, it seems hard to fathom from where 'trivial' complaints come to pester GPs unnecessarily. (1) The emphasis throughout is on not <u>bothering</u> or <u>worrying</u> the doctor, and only calling on her/his services when absolutely necessary.

These views reflect the respondents' feelings about 'proper cause'. The tendency only to visit GPs when forced because of severe impairment, discomfort or disruption of everyday life obviously affects the rate at which people use GPs services. The nature of the populations from which these respondents are drawn (largely working class council tenants) means that they are thought to use such services more than the average in Britain.(2) It also means that use is a poor indicator of need for health care because individuals are deferring visits and treating conditions themselves. Their perceived needs reflected in these practices will go unnoticed by policy-makers who usually rely on utilisation rates.

People comment on the structures of the GP service and the personal qualities of particular doctors. The structure of the service consists of several separate things. For most people, the waiting room is important because patients often have to wait a long time. Those who are satisfied with the waiting rooms at their GP's surgeries pass few comments about them, but others complain a great deal:

Maria (MG): There's hard wooden seats and everybody's too close together, spreading germs.

Janet (PH): Oh it's bad. Not very comfortable and it's old fashioned.

Mick (DW): It's a pokey hole.

Don (DW): It's damn cold... Not comfortable.

Most hope that the surgeries themselves are well-equipped and up-to-date, feeling unable and unqualified to comment with any certainty.

The type of practice provoked many comments, particularly concerning the number of doctors present. There is no overall agreement over a preference for single-handed or group systems, with people offering positive and negative views about both types. Those who prefer a single doctor usually refer to traditional 'family practitioners':

Alix (MG): One on his own. You get to know him, to talk to him. You feel better to go and ask him for advice.

Pat (DW): On his own because you find you see one doctor, and then if you go back, you have to see another doctor and then he says different things and you can get confused.

Leslie (PH): You get more personal treatment.

Some emphasise that they like to see a particular doctor in a group practice, one whom they trust or know:

Sandra (DW): I prefer to see my own doctor. I don't think the other doctors really know you, even though they're in the same group.

Others stress the importance of second opinions or the ease of seeing a doctor, any doctor, in a group practice:

Arthur (MG): I prefer the group. You can have a second or third opinion then. It's very good.

Betty (MG): I'd sooner have a group because you've got better choice. I mean, doctors are only human beings like us and they can be taken ill.

Fred (DW): Partnership, as they are now, you can always go in, anytime. You can book with any of them.

David (PH): You've got more chance of seeing one and... four can chew over the facts amongst themselves and come up with different ideas.

Group practices were the most common amongst the respondents, all of whom were registered with a GP on the NHS. Most seemed content with the sort of practice they had, or just accepted it:

Edith (DW): I don't mind as long as he's a good doctor and I can get on with him all right.

Gordon (PH): Well, if I've got faith in them, I don't care who it is.

Joyce (PH): I don't mind as long as I see somebody and they're helpful.

The most common source of complaints lies in the organisation of the practice, particularly in waiting times, making appointments, calling doctors out:

Louise (AC): I don't like to go to surgery, and I don't go very often. When you go there, it is a waste of time. So many. For me to go there, it is very important. We have to sit and wait for your turn - ages you have to wait.

Steph (MG): My husband went a week ago and he had to wait ten days [for an appointment]. He wanted to go after work and the doctor that week was doing mornings, so he had to wait.

Gordon (PH): You sometimes have a lot of 'bovver' getting through to them on the 'phone... He doesn't appear to be open all that long in the day - about four hours.

Leslie (PH): It's diabolical! Two hours sitting about in a bloody surgery - especially when you're not well.

Elaine (MG): My husband had an ulcer operation and in the night he had a coughing fit and all the stitches burst open... I called the number and they put me through to some number in the city and they said, 'don't worry, he won't bleed to death'... That was three am. I waited and waited. They didn't come until 8 o'clock. I think that's terrible.

Mary (DW): When the children have things like chickenpox, the doctors don't like coming out... They haven't got the bedside manner as the old doctors used to have. After six o'clock they're off duty. They go onto this emergency system whereas the old doctors used to be on all the time.

The question of time emerges as one of the most important. Patients dislike waiting too long for their consultation and they expect to be given a reasonable amount of time with the doctor. Those doctors who give enough time are praised; those who do not are critised:

Frank (PH): We're prepared to put ourselves out to see Dr. Wallace. He always listens to you.

Eleanor (MG): Yes, he's nice. He has the time to talk and he explains things and draws diagrams.

Bernard (MG): The one I've got, he's very good, he keeps you there for 10-15 minutes and listens to you.

Vanessa (MG): I think they should give you more time. It's just, you tell them what's wrong and they write it down and that's it, get out. They ought to spend more time, go into detail.

Danny (AC): I don't often see the doctor. I haven't really got time... It's just 'What's the matter?' A swift exam, tablets and away.

Earl (AC): They don't seem to take an interest in what you've got. It's just 'Oh, you've got this, I'll give you so many pills to take'... If the doctor doesn't have proper contact with the patient, there's no point in going... They could spend more time with the patient, break down the problem easier, diagnose it better... You're in and out before you've had a chance to tell him what's wrong... Doctors should be more versatile, visit people in their homes, see the conditions they're living in, what kind of stresses they're under.

Gareth (PH): They hurry you. He's writing out a

prescription before I've said anything... They don't spend time to see what is actually wrong with you.

The respondents' comments about the amount of time doctors allow them are closely linked with their opinions about the doctor's personal qualities. Studies have posited that patients' perceptions of doctors' personalities and affective behaviour may be <u>the</u> most important factor leading to patient compliance or co-operation.(3) A doctor's personal qualities are certainly closely scrutinised by most and judgements on their competence may be made on these criteria. Whilst the doctor's medical knowledge and expertise may not be within the lay person's judgement, her/his personality clearly is:

Ray (PH): I've only had one occasion to visit him and I was extremely satisfied with the treatment I got. He was polite and pleasant... He treated me with the utmost respect.

Dennis (DW): I switched my doctors and I've been a lot better since... He does a lot better for me. He make me feel comfortable.

Julie (DW): He knows I tend to be a worrier... He's good because he knows what I'm like. He will examine me. He will sit and listen.

Sufiya (AS): She listens to the patient very well and you feel psychologically better when you talk to her. Half your illness is gone when you talk to her because she is very nice, very friendly and speaks Punjabi.

Donna (AC): You go in and say this is wrong and then she'll start writing straight away. She never looks at you... She don't explain. Like they say all these words and they don't tell you exactly what it means.

Marian (PH): He's a very good doctor... very caring. Not ready to just write out a prescription, and he reads your notes before-hand.

Keith (PH): It's a bus-ride away but it's well worth going. I wouldn't change him for the world... He's the best.

A minority criticise the doctors because they are Asian. May, Tom, Vera and Jack of Deanswood make brief racist comments; others go into greater detail:

Michelle (MG): Well, he's a darkie, so he's hard to understand sometimes.

Leslie (PH): I don't like them at all... It's crazy up there. It's ridiculous. I mean, they're all bloody Asians, they can't understand a word you're talking about.

Lilian (PH): We haven't got British trained doctors,

right? We have got Indian doctors, right? And I don't think that the way they talk you can go and talk to your doctor... I don't think they really understand us.

It is among the respondents from London that the most dissatisfaction is felt. In London, more than one-half have specific complaints about their GPs. Some of their comments have already been mentioned; a few others follow:

Leroy (AC): She's (GP) controlling it [the consultation]. When I go in I feel shy and I don't speak up and say what's wrong, what I think is wrong. She asks questions and I just answer them. Then she scribbles out a thing for you... I come out of the doctor's, I look at it, and, 'What am I suffering from?'... You always know she's the doctor, and you're like, like a little kid.

Claire (PH): I've just given up. I've really had bad experiences since last May with doctors. The illness is continuous and you're rushed in and rushed out and I was left for so long that the infection in my stomach really multiplied - ovaries, fallopian tubes. In the end, we had to call an emergency doctor in and he sent me straight to hospital and said I should've been in there weeks ago... I haven't got any confidence at all in doctors.

Roger (PH): I showed him my foot the other weekend it was swollen and the doctor didn't really want to look at it. You know, 'Yeah, yeah'.

Taresh (AS): Every time I tell her I am not having proper periods, she says 'Go for the test, you might be pregnant.' But I am not. Every time she says this, even though I have got the coil.

In the other areas, complaints are much less common. In Deanswood most people are satisfied; some are delighted:

Jack (DW): I can't criticise the health centre when it is the most up-to-date place there is in the city. It's like a mini-hospital.

Nick (DW): We've got the best possible doctor and I'm completely satisfied.

In Mossley green, there is a mixture of opinions, with the majority being apathetically satisfied with what they have and a few being clearly critical.

In London, the criticisms are compounded by the lack of choice over practitioners because of closed lists:

Dora (PH): When we first came here, I went up the road and the receptionist said, 'Oh no, we can't take any more.' I was told that was because of our age.

Marian (PH): That one only took people in his area and

he was fully booked; couldn't fit me in, but when I got
pregnant with the first, because I was pregnant, he felt
I needed a doctor and as I refused to go to the others,
he took me on.

Clare (PH): I did not want to change my doctor, but I
couldn't get on to the doctor's books that I wanted to
change to. It's fully booked now.

In assessing their GPs, then, people take into consideration
a number of criteria. One of the most important of these is
for the doctor to be nice, to listen to what they want to say,
and to give them what they consider to be enough time. They
expect the doctor to tell them what is wrong and help them to
cope with it. Some are lucky in having the 'ideal' doctor;
others expect the ideal but have to put up with less. People
expect to be told the diagnosis and the reason for treatment -
why else do they refer themselves to the formal health care
system? - but often they emerge from the consultation without
a clear picture. The easiest way to restore the balance and
regain control is for them to criticise their doctor or
doctors in general. People who are very dissatisfied with
their GPs do not always return, but they have few other places
to which they can turn. Only a few, as we have seen, go to
alternative practitioners. Many find it difficult to go to
a doctor and just submit - they want to say what is wrong with
them, but the aura of the medical profession, the structure
of the consultation and often the attitude of the doctor
militate against the patient being forthcoming:

Martha (AC): Doctors see health in one way _their_ way,
because they have been trained for that. Like when you
go to the doctor and you have a common cold and they give
you medicine and say you have a touch of bronchitis...
They are only just looking at it as to what is written in
the book... People often know what is wrong with them,
but you can't tell the doctor because he don't want you
to tell him his job... I think they should listen more.

DRUGS

As Martha indicates, another common criticism of doctors is
that they over-prescribe and give what are regarded as
unsuitable or ineffective drugs. On the whole, people are
reluctant to take drugs of any sort:

Fred (DW): I don't like taking any of them to be
truthful. If I have a headache or owt like that I shake
it off without anything.

Dennis (DW): I don't like messing about with drugs and
things... I've been taking them a long time now, a long
period and I'm getting to rely on them. I don't want it
to be habit-forming.

Miriam (MG): I'm not one for taking tablets or anything.
I don't believe in it unless I'm _ill_.

Carlton (AC): I will only take a tablet if I'm really bad, bad, bad, bad, bad!... Don't like putting them down my system... I'd rather trust something from my mum than from a doctor, even if I was dying.

Many people admit to taking a lower dose than that prescribed by their GPs.

Clare (PH): He said, 'Did you taken the [Valium]' And I said, 'No, but the toilet went well on them!' I didn't need them.

Emily (AC): I take iron, folic acid and ascorbic acid tablets. I've been taking one a day, but really I should take three a day, like I did when I came from hospital.

Joe (AC): Sometimes I take them and sometimes I don't... As long as I can get to work for Monday morning, that's all right.

Eleanor (MG): I am supposed to take intel [inhaler] three times a day, but I just take it when I've got the tightness... It would be far too much money to keep taking everything. It's the same with the [eczema] oil. I use it so sparingly because it's just a luxury. I go out and buy handcream instead, but this oil is specially for my condition.

Maureen (DW): I took [stomach medicine] last night. I don't take it as prescribed, I take it as I need it. I'm supposed to take it before meals, but some days I find it's better than others.

Geeta (AS): (The doctor) said I needed the iron tablets... He told me to take three tablets a day, but I am taking only one. I feel too hot with three - like hot flushes. They don't agree with me.

Geeta is not the only one to raise the subject of side-effects from prescribed drugs:

Don (DW): Thyroid I have to take for the rest of my life. And angina, myxoedema and water. They're the only things that help me. If I take three a day, I might get cramp - a side effect.

Tasneem (AS): In our country, they think that herbal treatment is cool and soothing, there are not side effects, but the medicines, they are hot, they are not very good, they can give you side-effects due to the chemicals in them. Herbs, on the other hand, they are natural things. Even if they don't give you good effects, they won't give you any bad effects.

Dorothy (DW): The tablets have been more trouble than the [uveitis]... If I cut myself, I don't heal properly for about eight weeks...

They [steroids] are all right at first when you put on weight and you've got more energy... It's difficult to come off them. Some days I shake and I can't be bothered. And I've lost a lot of weight. I wouldn't advise anyone to go on them.

Frank (PH): I don't like taking drugs because I think they all have side effects.

Eleanor (MG): I came off the pill because of that big scare about it being carcinogenic.

Most people in Britain are used to having tablets prescribed and so do not object to them:

Brenda (PG): I don't like taking either [tablets or medicine], but if I've got to, I'd rather take tablets.

Those of Afro-Caribbean descent, however, especially those who have migrated in the last twenty years, remember taking liquid preparations, medicines, during their childhoods. They do not like taking tablets, do not always believe they will work, and bemoan the lack of medicines available in Britain:

Delores (AC): Whatever sickness you get, it is in the blood. What water would do, where water would wash, a tablet can't do. A tablet has to dissolve before it can do the trick, but if you take a glass of medicine, it means it goes through the body. If you're lying down, you can feel it.

Ruby (AC): Back home they give you medicine, not pills. Real medicine... I can't take capsules - they make me sick... You feel the medicine working more than you feel the pills.

Earl (AC): At least in liquid form, you can see some form of what you are taking. In tablet form, it could be anything.

HOSPITALS

For complaints that cannot be dealt with by lay coping strategies or GP prescriptions and treatment, hospitals may be used. They can also be used for accidents or in emergencies. In fact, almost everyone has experienced some sort of hospital treatment. These experiences are the basis for people's opinions about how satisfactory the treatment was. People also take into account the local reputation of the hospital, gleaned from many people's experiences. Those who have had particularly good or unpleasant episodes of treatment tend to tell the story of the particular circumstances. Others talk in the abstract or extrapolate particular experiences to generalise about all hospital matters. Again there were some areal differences. Those from Deanswood tended to praise hospitals whereas those in Parkheath were much more critical. People from Mossley Green were less definite in their opinions.

Most of those who praise the hospitals speak of their good reputations:

> Jack (DW): At 'the Paddock'. You have a team of doctors and nurses... what flies all over the world if there is anybody important in another country what's really ill...the top people they are to perform operations on all these big wigs abroad.

> Geoff (DW): I think in this city they're fantastic for hospitals. I mean, we must be one of the best cities, not just in this country but in the world for hospitals. It's renowned for hospitals... 'St. Thomas's' - one of the finest heart hospitals...and the university for general diseases.

> Michelle (MG): You have to go to the city for the big major hospitals, really, although 'St. Margarets' is fairly good, you know, they have got everything emergency wise, and 'the District'. You could always do with more, but what town couldn't? You know they'll do a good job.

Others base their praise on their (good) experiences of treatment. Sometimes the personal qualities of the doctor again become important:

> Doreen (PH): The most marvellous treatment I had. I haven't got anything to complain about.

> Nick (DW): I've been in 'the Cross' and the 'Paddock'. What I can remember, I got the best treatment possible.

> Wendy (MG): When (son with Down's syndrome) was born, 'the District' were marvellous, absolutely marvellous... I am very, very happy with the health services, even the ambulance service round here is first class... I think people in Mossley don't know how lucky they are.

> Dolores (AC): Great! I 'll always praise the doctors and nurses.

> Rani (AS): They treated me very well... They brought me an interpreter... and she explained everything.

Some people are willing to praise hospitals openly, but often, if the treatment is good or adequate, people accept it and do not find it necessary to be overly grateful. Poor treatment, however, by its very nature, encourages people to complain loudly. As we have seen with GPs, people criticise unexpected behaviour or perceived inadequate treatment in order to make sense of it and to restore their control over the situation. There are more critical stories, then, than praiseworthy ones, but by far the majority of people are satisfied with the hospitals they attend and/or visit. As with positive stories, the criticisms divide easily into two: those that decry hospitals in general or particular hospitals because of reputation; and those who feel they have had very poor treatment indeed. We think it is worth examining some of these 'horror' stories in detail so that practitioners and policy-makers may have some sense of what it is like to be on the receiving end of poor treatment and to show how often simple explanations or a few minutes of discussion to gain the patients' co-operation may have avoided or alleviated many of the problems.

There are a lot of criticisms about waiting times - both on lists and actually at out - and in-patients' departments:

Gordon (PH): Whenever you go, you always have to hang about half the day.

Alec (PH): My wife waited 18 months to have her veins done. That is a bloody long time.

Len (MG): The doctor said that it is a long waiting list... When you have paid into the health service from when you were 14 to 48 and you have had nothing out of it, well, all right, I have been lucky, but when you want something out of it, you can't get anything.

Donna (AC): Talking about other people's experiences, I don't think it's all that good. You go along and you have to wait a long time. You could be bleeding, you still have to wait for someone to see you.

Some complain that the doctors are not friendly enough, are too rushed, cannot explain things, or are rude:

Peter (MG): I don't rate 'St. Margaret's'... My sister went in to have bunions done and he ruined her feet... He turned round and told her, 'This is not a beauty parlour, it's a hospital. We've done the best we can for you. You are dismissed'.

Carlton (AC): I had to go back every first of the month for an injection... 'Hello, come in' Woomph! Didn't tell me what they was doing, what they were for. Nothing. You've just going in like a dummy. You don't know what's going on.

Pat (DW): They dragged me in about eight weeks before I had (son) and told me I was having a very small baby, about two-and-a-half pounds. They wouldn't tell me anything else... I signed myself out of hospital because I just wasn't satisfied... [Two days later] I haemorrhaged - placenta praevia - breech. They must have known. If they'd said I'd have stayed in ... If they'd explained to me, I would've stayed... They would explain. It's my body they're going to mess around with.

James (DW): We think the handicapped are poorly looked after... Carol (daughter) came home with about 30 lacerations on her arm and we've had this three times before. We got onto them and contacted the police... I had to let them know things like this can't happen.

Millie (AC): [The 'Blue ribband' hospital] is useless. Damn useless. They are doing big, big research. They haven't got time for me, for headaches. If you go in with your small, small, disease, you will die there.

Peter (MG): We had a doctor who explained why dad died...but I just stood there, 'Yeah yeah'. But he couldn't explain. He tried, but he couldn't tell me. I tried to talk to him. The nurse tried to help us, explain in our words, like. That's the way they are, I suppose.

Naseem (AS): They couldn't find anything wrong with my back. The doctor kept saying I was making too much fuss about nothing. That was Dr. Buckle, he said that we people should all be called - that I should be called Mrs. Brown because of my colour... Lots of people say it happens to them as well.

The cuts in services over the last few years also provoked critical remarks. People are worried that the loss of services will affect their chances of getting good treatment and lengthen the waiting lists:

David (PH): What's the use of having a hospital if you can't go there in an emergency?

Arthur (MG): It's all very well for those who live on the other side of Mossley. I can't get on an off a 'bus easily. It's too far... They should've built the new one up here.

Stuart (MG): There's plenty of hospitals, but there's a shortage of staff. There's a couple of wards closed down and beds lying empty.

Geoff (DW): There's a lot of waiting lists for people that need care and attention... Since the cutbacks in the NHS well there's more waiting lists.

Finally, we turn to a sample of the 'horror' stories - the tales people told of very bad treatment and about which they were very angry, bitter, and upset. Again it is interesting to focus on a time during the story when a straight forward explanation or request for the patient's permission might have improved the situation, or at least made matters more bearable and/or comprehensible:

Tasneem (AS): They thought there some trouble between me and my husband... They asked if I was happy with my husband [They were married by arrangement]... They took blood tests and X-rays but they couldn't find any illness at all. After six months they said there was nothing wrong with me... Then I started to get a temperature, very high temperature and it went on for a month. One night I felt a very, very severe pain in my chest and my husband had to call the doctor... He came and said I've got an attack of pneumonia so he sent me straight away to [an isolation unit]... They took more x-rays and said I'd got pleurisy, fluid on the lungs. I must've had this all along... The doctor said I'd been having this trouble for more than a year. They should've found out earlier... They had X-rays of the whole family. At that time they were concerned because they knew it was due to them the trouble had become worse... I caught TB, you see.

Initially, Rajinda (AS) said that the death of her daughter occurred because, 'she missed her daddy very much and she got a high temperature and chickenpox and complications caused her death'. But this was not the end of her story:

Rajinda (AS): When she was young, she had the whooping cough vaccine and it damaged her brain. She was not talking until she was two and she could not balance her head at all. Over here, I was taking her to every clinic and they never told us she had any brain damage, but when we went to India, a consultant professor told me her brain was affected due to that injection... They didn't tell us at all. Sometimes they pay damages, but they wouldn't ever tell us. She was six months old when we found out about the damage and we stopped going to our family doctor because he hadn't told us... The injection was done here when she was three months old, and they got a signature from us to say that if anything happened from this injection, they are not responsible... The people at the clinic said it was not their fault, that she was brain damaged at birth, not by the injection, but the hospital said she was perfect when she was born... so, instead of doing everything for her, they never even agreed it was their fault.

Naseem (AS): [The delivery of the twins] was forceps and I was three days in labour pain. It was a bad one and they gave me stitches... The stitches got septic and they left the after-birth in... When I came round, I just said, 'pain, pain', and they ignored me. Then when they saw I was all swollen they took me to the theatre and, without anaesthetic, they did the D & C [dilation and curettage]. It was so painful. Afterwards they were not helpful, either. They gave me some tablets for the milk. They didn't tell me what they were for. They have given me all the lumps in my breasts... They aren't very helpful with the Asian ladies... They upset me and I'm sure they are worse with the other ladies [Naseem speaks perfect English, unlike many of the other women].

Roger (PH): Three years ago, I went in for a vasectomy and I ended up in there for six weeks... They blew a hole in my throat and I had a collapsed right lung and I had pneumonia set in, through the anaesthetist's fault... They've admitted liability to it... I nearly died in there. Ever since then, I've been suffering - like infections and everything else. I've got asthma now which I never had when I was a child. I had to pack in my job because of my health... (my wife) lost all her hair, all through what happened... What happened to me, I wouldn't wish it on anybody. Whatever compensation we got out of this, it won't be worth anything of what I've lost. My health and my job... Normally, the health service is good. All right, I was unfortunate they made a mistake with my operation... You can never get another health, can you? Once you've lost it, you've had it.

Ray (PH): Twelve years ago, I had a urine infection. They gave me a cystoscopy and I finished up in there for three weeks. A slipped disc blew up while I was in there, so they put me on traction and I got catheta fever (sic)... It was a lot worse than I expected.

Taresh (AS): My daughter, when she was born became very ill. She had diarrhoea and vomiting and she was not taking any milk at all, and the nurses, they were getting angry. They were saying that I was just pretending she wasn't getting any milk, that she was not sick at all but that I was a greedy mother... [After an operation on the hand] When I came round I felt sick... One nurse was very mad and angry. She said, 'Why are you being sick and saying you feel dizzy and this and that? Nothing is happening to you. You are pretending that you are being sick. You are making yourself sick.'

Millie's interview consisted almost solely of problems at the hospital. She tells of neglect and abuse after the birth.

Most people in Britain are used to having tablets prescribed and so do not object to them:

Millie (AC): When I was in hospital, they ask me if I want family planning. I say 'yes'. When I went to the post-natal clinic, well they fitted me with this coil - they supposed to check me up, but they didn't check, just fix me a coil. When she was doing it, I didn't know what she was doing. I thought she was examining me or something. When she finish, she said, 'I have fixed you a beautiful coil'. And I say, 'WHAT!' I shout, 'After six weeks? That ain't right.'... She says, 'It's beautiful.' I say, 'It don't bother me whether it's beautiful or not, I come for a check up.'

Millie confirms throughout that the coil was inserted without her knowledge, let alone her permission, and that the doctors were inconsiderate and ignorant of her preferences:

Millie (AC): Back home [Ghana], when you have a baby, you don't sleep with a man for maybe three to six months. But here, after three or four weeks they do back to their husbands. We don't do that. I was waiting until three or four months when I know I'm fit to sleep with a man...

... Since then, whenever I see my period, I get pain. I
get pain. Never in my life did I have period pain... So,
I went to 'Blue Ribband' Hospital. So they take it [the
coil] out and fix me with another one. I say, 'I don't
want another one,' but they already fix it. Because I
always use 'Miss', because I am not married, so they think
they have a right to do what they did... Explain! No!
They fix me before they explain.

Millie's story continues that the second contraceptive coil
caused as many problems as the first. She was eventually
rushed into hospital after collapsing in pain and fibroids
were diagnosed. She was advised to have a total hysterectomy
and she agreed to it at the age of 33 years to be rid of the
pain she was suffering. Millie believes strongly that it was
the contraceptive coil that caused the growth of fibroids and
ultimately her hysterectomy. She is understandably bitter
about her experiences and feels she was treated in the way she
was because she is a single, black parent.

It is important to note that many of the episodes of
perceived poor treatment reported above occur in London and
to the black respondents. For Londoners, it would seem that
being close to a world famous hospital does not ensure that
you will get good or even adequate treatment for relatively
common or minor complaints. For the black respondents, there
is also the every-present hazard of racism, conscious or
unconscious, which may result in much worse treatment for them
than white patients. Some of the stories above can be clearly
related to racist attitudes on the part of hospital staff:
Tasneem being told her chest trouble was caused by her
supposedly unhappy arranged marriage; Naseem and Taresh being
ignored when they were in considerable pain; and Millie
receiving a contraceptive coil without her permission because
she is a single, black mother and is a carrier of sickle-cell
trait.(4)

The 'horror' stories also challenge the idea that patients
do not want to know what is wrong with them or what has gone
awry. Some doctors' paternalistic attitudes that they know
best and that patients are better off not knowing,(5) are not
borne out. People do want to know what is·happening to them,
but they want it explained in plain terms, not jargon.
Several of the stories may not have been so horrific had a
member of medical staff taken the time to talk to the patient
and offer explanation (see the stories of Peter, Pat, Rajinda,
Naseem) or ask permission (Millie's case).

PRIVATE TREATMENT

The complaints about NHS treatment voiced amongst the London
respondents are also reflected in their views about private
treatment. More than one half of those from Parkheath say
they would consider using private doctors, compared with less
than one third in the other areas. Their reasons are mainly
that private treatment is quicker, but also that they may give
'better' drugs, devote more time and be more careful.

Marian (PH): My mother has to have her toe cut off... We have to wait 8 months to have that done. I asked to have it done privately and it's 200 pounds.

Mary (DW): I had no use of this arm and I was given an eight month's appointment... and we said, 'Right, we'll go private.' Got in the next day. It's wrong.

Ivy (AC): You're paying out and you <u>expect</u> to get your money's worth... The drugs are much stronger than the NHS because you pay more money.

Ruby (AC): They give you something different than the national doctor would give, and sometimes they give you more. You have to keep going back to the national doctor, but sometimes the private doctor will give you an injection and that cures it.

Lilian (PH): If you are paying for a doctor, you are going to get a doctor that is going to be interested, aren't you?

Not many people have actually made use of private doctors. It may be that the expressed preference of one half of those in Parkheath and a third each in Deanswood and Mossley Green may stem from the changing nature of British society which has imposed individualistic, choice-oriented attitudes on sections of the British Public (see chapter 1) and cut the NHS to the extent that people feel forced to consider alternatives when faced with appointments far into the future.(6)

The private system offers an alternative which is not always out of the each of ordinary people, most of whom would put their health at the top of their priorities:

Claire (PH): Dr. Simmonds, he's a psychiatrist and a homeopathic doctor. He spent nearly two hours with me, when through case history, listened, put over his point and I've got a lot more confidence in him... 30 pounds for the first consultation with treatment and tablets. I've got to go back in a fortnight and that is 18 pounds consultation and tablets... I'd rather pay and get the attention and ask questions and not get ushered out than take a tranquilizer... I'm intelligent, I don't need sedatives. I need help to get to the main problem.

Ian (MG): I may like to go into hospital private. It's quicker... I had a vasectomy ten years ago and that was private. The GP put me in touch with the specialist.

Tansneem (AS): Sometimes my family doctor doesn't give so much medicine for the children, so I, for my own satisfaction, just call the private doctor, he only charges 3 pounds for a visit and then gives a prescription.

There are still some people, however, who will refuse to use private treatment on principle, and who are strongly against the conservative government's policies. Most of these come from the areas of West Yorkshire and the West Midlands, although there are a few from the South East:

> Maureen (DW): They're doing the two wards up now and we're a nationalised hospital but we've got BUPA nurses and two of the doctors have bought this wing that's being done up under the national health... We have got a beautiful new entrance - who the hell sees it? Nobody!... What use is an entrance when the wards want seeing to?... The people who run the NHS don't run it properly. They don't run it for the patients, they run it as a business.

> Alex (PH): I prefer the national health... I disagree with this privatisation, definitely. They get enough money, they should use it wisely.

> Betty (MG): I would sooner have the national health service myself and not private. I mean, not everybody is in that position where they can have a private doctor and there again, they only get the same treatment as the national health.

> Ron (DW): I don't think that there's any difference. I don't think that paying money's going to make any difference.

Many also think that they could not afford private treatment, and for those who have good GPs and pleasant experiences of hospital treatment, why bother?

> Doreen (PH): I don't think I could get better treatment.

> Doris (MG): I like the national health.

> Rupe (DW): I'm all right with the national health.

One reason for bothering could be the perceived deterioration in the service that the NHS can offer. People are pessimistic for the future of a state health system:

> Alec (PH): This national health, I don't go much on. When it first came into operation it was a good thing, but this day and age, this government is proceeding towards private hospitals... Everything she [Mrs. Thatcher] said, she's gone against... I don't think there'll be a national health in a few months' time.

> Ivy (AC): Improvements? What a chance when Maggie Thatcher's cutting down on the health service so you're not even sure of getting the right treatment these days.

CONCLUSIONS

These cuts also illustrate the individual's apparent

powerlessness to control or change her/his way of life and the way things are. In the consideration of the formal health care system, we see the seeming dominance of the medical profession and administrators who are beyond individual control and sometimes comprehension. They establish the parameters of daily life in the clinic or hospital. We all use our experiences and perceptions to construct the personal and social worlds in which we live, but the experiences and perceptions of some are more important and powerful than others. The forces that shape life in Britain (see chapters 1 and 4) are those that, in the main, fashion the nature of the formal health care system. These are medical practice and definitions, closely allied to the dominant economic and political ways of thinking and acting.

As this chapter has shown, however, people do not simply acquiesce to these forces. They may often feel resigned and/or demoralised. Indeed, as Berger and Luckmann have expressed it: "He (sic) who has the bigger stick has the better chance of imposing his definition of reality."(7) But we do not have to stand there and be beaten. People's own definitions of reality - particularly through expressed dissatisfactions - will alter the relationships that exist in the world, although the outcome of such negotiation in terms of, say, the nature and quality of health services provided will largely depend on its economic and political context, to which fatalism, acquiescence and resignation are but individual reactions.

People expressed dissatisfactions about doctors, drugs and hospital treatment. Eventually, they modify the definitions of medical practice established by the medical profession. They begin to challenge, though increasing awareness of the damage wrought by public expenditure cuts to the health service, the political order. They help to make people less acquiescent. This may provide a basis for change, but it may not. Unfortunately, many of the expressed dissatisfactions and criticisms are based on and directed at specific instances and services. Where they are generalised, it is usually in terms of what is wrong with the health service not the economic and political climate in Britain. If individuals are resigned to the ways things are, there seems to be little basis for effecting social change. We address some of these issues of acquiescence in the final chapter, in which we also return to the themes of policy and method first addressed in chapters 1 and 2.

FOOTNOTES

1. Studies of GPs show that they complain that around one quarter of all consultations are 'trivial.' In other words, they are treatable by the patient or unimportant: a waste of medical time. There is then a serious difference between lay and medical opinion, a view suggested by R. Fitzpatrick, The experience of illness, Tavistock, 1984. For the studies, see A. Cartwright, Patients and their doctors, RKP 1967 and A. Cartwright and R. Anderson, General practice revisited, Tavistock, 1981.

2. See Office of Population Censuses and Surveys, General household survey, H.M.S.O., 1984; J. Eyles and J. Donovan, Regional variations in perceptions and experiences of health and health care, End of Research Report to ESRC 1986.

3. See, for example, T. Garrity, Medical compliance, Social Science and Medicine, 15E, 1981, 215-22; M. Calnan, Clinical uncertainty, Sociology of Health and Illness, 6, 1984, 74-85.

4. Carrying sickle-cell trait is thought to cause no ill effects. When two carriers have children, however, there is a one-in-four chance that each child will get the life-threatening sickle-cell anaemia (Millie's son has this). Sickle-cell anaemia causes red blood cells to become sickle shaped, and if the individual exercises, they can cause episodes of severe pain, known as crises. The disease has many complications and is incurable. Life expectancy is short. It is now possible to detect the disease in a foetus and abortions can·be considered, but in the U.S., calls for such abortions without adequate counselling have provoked charges of genocide. See B. Konotey - Ahulu, The Guardian 8th January, 1982.

5. This attitude is certainly not outmoded but has recently been documented by J. Todd, Cruel absurdity of telling your patients everything, Doctor, 15, 1985, p. 37.

6. Changes in the private sector are documented in annual surveys in The Financial Times.

7. P. Berger and T. Luckmann, The social construction of reality Penguin, 1967.

7 Health research and questions of method and policy

HEALTH RESEARCH, REGIONAL DIFFERENCES AND POLICY

In this final chapter, we begin by summarising some of the main findings of our study. We discovered that people had difficulty in defining 'health'. While health tended to be seen as deteriorating with age, it was mainly related to other aspects of life, usually work, family responsibilities or functional capacity in general. This definition in fact is linked to the ways in which illness is perceived. Illness is the disruption of routine. It is inevitable, although even then some illnesses are considered to be more 'real' in their effects than others. It is only when the complaint is a real illness that most people see themselves as having 'proper cause' to use the formal health care system. Otherwise, 'minor' illnesses are ignored, worked through or treated with home remedies or proprietary drugs. Illness is then fully embedded in their daily activities. In a sense, a balance is achieved between what is felt (the illness) and what needs doing (work, family and so on). This means that many, even serious, complaints are defined away and the people suffering from these complaints considered themselves to be healthy, given their individual attributes and circumstances. Level of health changes with these circumstances. Illness is, therefore, a matter for negotiation as well as a physical characteristic. It has social meaning as well as objective definition - an important difference reflected in lay and medical beliefs (see chapter 2). It is illness that is important to people in their daily lives. Health, although sought by all, is a residual category. Illness is experienced; health merely taken-for-granted.

The meanings of health and illness are negotiated. This negotiation occurs with respect to individual circumstances and how these circumstances compare with necessary tasks and other people. These comparisons are also important in assigning causes to particular episodes of illness,their being used in determining to whom sympathy and understanding should be given. Some illnesses are considered to be trivial, avoidable or matters of life style (and therefore choice). In these cases, sympathy may be withdrawn or withheld. These illnesses are those without due or proper cause and the label hypochondriac may be applied to particular individuals. In other circumstances, worry is thought to be a significant and unavoidable cause of ill-health. Other important causes include luck, chance and loneliness, the last-named being linked to worry, depression and stress. Loneliness particulary affects those of Asian descent as they compare their present lies with the past in other places. This is in fact one of the few exceptions to the widely held views of health and illness. There seems to be a medicalised culture shared by the vast majority of our respondents (see also chapter 2).

This culture suggests that regional consciousnesses with respect to health and illness do not exist. But it is not as straightforward as that. While undoubtedly there is this shared view of the world,there are exceptions. We of course can say nothing about class variations but there are some subcultural and locational differences, these being largely based on the material circumstances of the particular subcultures and localities. For example, racism imposes on black people particular disadvantages which affect their quality of life and health. But their different cultural heritages provide different ways of seeing and acting in the world. Those of Asian descent, for example, retain some traditional views of health, illness and body function,namely those of hot and cold. They do not share, then, completely this medicalised culture, although there are signs that they are increasingly absorbing these ideas. Those of Afro-Caribbean descent have also retained and passed on some traditional ideas. These differ in that they are not so much concerned with cause as with coping, by providing home remedies.

Living in a particular place also has its consequences, as it determines the nature of environment and work. Those living in Deanswood and Mossley Green saw themselves as living in good or improving housing conditions and in areas where pollution was becoming less of a problem than in the past. But for work, the situation was deteriorating. Almost the opposites applied to those living in London (both in Parkheath and among the black respondents). Work was fairly plentiful but the quality of housing and environment were seen as worsening. These circumstances may be explained by the uneven development of Britain over the last ten years, which have seen an expansion in the South East at the expense of much of the rest of the country. This material context also has consequences for people's attitudes and senses of well-being. These emerge as a pessimism and demoralisation, important dimensions of regional consciousness in modern Britain. In London rather than there being an overt pessimism, there is complaint and rancour when things do not seem right. For example, there was greater dissatisfaction with the quality of the health service in Parkheath than elsewhere. In the North in Deanswood, the decline in Britain's fortunes has been present for a long period and so it has become not so much accepted but absorbed. It is rather taken-for-granted. In the Midlands in Mossley Green, the decline has been more recent and from a level of greater prosperity. There is an acceptance of the ways things are which takes the form of acquiescence and demoralisation, while people are adjusting to these changes. An analogy may be drawn with the effects of depression on an individual. It takes time to come to terms with the complaint (the state of Mossley Green) but eventually an adjustment is made and the depression is absorbed and life returns to a different kind of 'normality' (Deanswood).

These portraits are of course overdrawn and probably time-specific. We have drawn attention to them to show the differences that can and do exist within an overarching medicalised and indeed national culture. They also demonstrate that how we feel is greatly dependent on what we are and do, in other words on the state of the nation and its local effects. These local differences also emerge in people's views of the formal health care system. Those in London (Parkheath and the black groups) are the most critical both of GPs and hospitals and they use private treatment to the greatest extent. In contrast, those in Deanswood are the most satisfied, while those in Mosely Green hold conflicting views. Of course within these regionally-based generalisations, there exist a wide range of personal experiences and therefore views. These individual perceptions and experiences make and yet modify the material contexts of the areas. In turn social and industrial structure, demographic characteristics and level and quality of service provision impinge on individual consciousness and well-being. In this way, we may see the relevance of resource allocation policies to shape and remould attitudes and perceptions. These policies are meant over time to equalise regional finance allocations on the basis of measured need for health care. But the starting-points for the exercise are extremely unequal, meaning that it is likely to take a long time to achieve the policy objective. Further, the measurement of need is inherently contestable so that there are likely to be conflicts over proposed and actual resource allocations. The picture is further complicated if we move from considering just the quantity of care and try to account for the quality of care in policy initiatives. There seems, for example, some relationships between waiting list size and timings (which seem at first sight to be related to the quantity of available resources e.g. number of specialist doctors, theatre nurses, operating rooms and so on) and good clinical practice.[1] Further, after reviewing the regional variations in avoidable deaths, Charlton and his colleagues concluded that "the extent of the unexplained variation in mortality warrants further investigation, since mortality from all of these diseases should be largely avoidable by efficient and effective health care... If it is established that there are indeed large variations in the quality of health care delivery from one part of the country to another this will have implications for resource allocation".(2) To recognise implications does not make remedial policies any more easy to implement. The difficulties inherent in altering resource allocation policies, especially in times of financial stringency or cost containment, to favour disadvantaged areas do not disappear. If little gets done when the experiences of individuals point to the obvious need for action,then the failure of policy will fuel the disillusion, frustration and resignation of those like we studied. Policy does not only allocate resources but also shapes consciousness. And as we shall see the forms of consciousness impinge on policy, especially in the form of health promotion and community care (the self-oriented policies). But we shall discuss these policies after we have established a broader context for policy-making and implementation in the 1980s and 1990s. But paradoxically, we can see the bases of this context in debates in the 1950s and 60s concerning the implications of resignation and acquiescence among working-class groups.

In the late 1950s and the 1960s there was debate in the social sciences concerning the acquiescence of the underprivileged in the inequalities to which they were and are subjected.(3) In later decades, the focus of debate shifted away from why individuals appear to acquiesce towards the structural features that produce the inequalities in the first place. In other words, attention moved for individual positions and perceptions to the mode of production and the failure of the state to alter significantly the material relations forged in the production process. While such a shift broadened the issues examined critically, it did have the unfortunate consequence of underemphasising the social position of individuals and groups (other than economic aggregates), as well as ideas and beliefs and from whence these derive. This ignoring of 'minds' was mirrored in political thought too, where the only serious investigation came from the New Right.

We shall return to political thought a little later. The early research on acquiescence focused on the apparent ignorance, habits and restricted expectations of the underprivileged. In his review of the literature, Runciman tried to go beyond these categories, although it must be noted that restricted expectations may simply be a realistic appraisal of what can be achieved in society given a particular starting point. This 'realism' meant that social discontents were kept at a relatively low level. In turn, the realism was based on the deprived selecting a point of reference in the social hierarchy that was fairly close to their present position. Aspirations and points of reference are, therefore, modified according to social position. As Runciman comments: "It may well be that the magnitude of the relative deprivations which are felt by the underprivileged is no greater than the magnitude of those felt by the very prosperous. The point is rather that whatever the relative magnitudes of relative deprivation, those near the bottom are likely, even in a society with an egalitarian ideology, to choose reference groups nearer the bottom than self-conscious egalitarianism would imply".(4) The deprived do not aim for rags-to-riches success but a decent standard of living, comparable with but not better than that enjoyed by the mass of citizens. It should be noted that deprivation is seen as a relative phenomenon (5) and that Runciman's point about magnitude of deprivation is supported by the British social attitudes report which shows that the scale of poverty in Britain is perceived to be greater among the well-off as opposed to the poor.(6) The poor are usually someone else whatever objective circumstances say.

Realistic and realisable expectations thus limit social discontents. A further limitation stems from how people see their expectations, however limited, being fulfilled. Up to the mid-1970s, there was a widespread, shared belief that a variable combination of individual effort and state aid would ensure that most people's expectations would be achieved and that, even if they continued to rise, future aspirations would also be so met. What has changed over the last ten years or so has been the climate in which those expectations are now worked out. (And with this we return to changes in political thought.) The years of the Conservative government have more than any other created a mood - a kind of populism which is assertive overseas and which stresses individual responsibility and provision, self-help and the family and freedom from state interference at home.(7) It is a mood and spirit of competitive individualism well-summarised in the words of Margaret Thatcher:

> The sense of being self-reliant, of playing a role within the family, of owning one's own property, of paying one's own way, are all part of the spiritual ballast which maintains responsible citizenship, and provides a solid foundation from which people look around to see what more they might do for others and for themselves.(8)

This 'spiritual ballast' has been extremely influential, especially as the psychic resistance to such ballast which might be mounted from working class values has been badly blunted by the assault from consumerist capitalism which we discussed in Chapter 1. In this framework, rights and entitlements (the satisfaction of expectations) become limited to those achieved through individual competitive effort. Welfare, for example, is not so much based on citizenship rights but more on contribution to the common good, with that good being narrowly defined in terms of economic, wealth and profit contribution. This has meant that the redistributions effected by the Conservatives have favoured the relatively well off, particularly through mortgage tax relief, the extensions to share ownership and the reduction of standard rates of tax. This kind of redistribution is also aided by the failure to index pensions, child benefit and long-term unemployment and sickness payments to increases in the cost of living. This is the material context which reinforces and is reinforced by the set of ideas now established. "What is needed", said Durkheim, "if social order is to reign is that the mass of men (sic) be content with their lot. But what is needed for them to be content, is not that they have more or less but that they be convinced that they have no right to more".(9) If they are so convinced, there are indeed few alternatives.

It is no coincidence that this convincing view, that there are few alternatives, has been accompanied by a fundamental shift in British society from what Loney calls a welfare society to a law-and-order society.(10) The emphasis on entitlement has shifted to one on social control. If the battle for minds looks as though it may be lost, then coercive action may be applied. The mood of competitive individualism is supported by a growing authoritarian state apparatus. Expenditure on social policy (housing in particular) and economic policy (especially regional aid and industrial investment assistance) has been decimated. But the level of public expenditure has not fallen. The social security budget has grown enormously to finance the victims of economic mismanagement. And so have the defence and police budgets.(11)

In other parts of health and welfare policy, there is encouragement of community and private practice and solutions. Social work has become increasingly prioritised because of limited resources. Statutory obligation in certain areas means that other clients become the responsibility of the 'community' in that they and their families and friends are left to fend for themselves. The role of the private sector for care of the elderly and handicapped in particular waits to be mapped out, although the growth in private residential homes has been vast. In health care, there has been encouragement of commercial medicine. We saw, amongst our respondents, how the presence of private medicine and its supposed advantages have received recognition and how NHS problems were seen as causes of dissatisfaction, worry and concern.

In general terms, then, policy emphasises more and more a self-cure strategy within a philosophy of cost containment. This was established by two government documents. The first stated that "the prime responsibility for his (sic) own health falls on the individual. The role of the health professions and of government is limited to ensuring that the public have access to such knowledge as is available about the importance of personal habit on health and at the very least, no obstacles are placed in the way of those who decide to act on the knowledge."(12) The second from the minister said that "I am sure you do not need reminding that the government's top priority must be to get the economy right; for that reason, it cannot be assumed that more money will always be available to be spent on health care."(13) This policy framework must be related to people's perceptions, expectations and aspirations as so much depends on individual action. If people are demoralised, resigned or acquiescent, it is probable that it will be difficult to motivate them to act. That difficulty may be then worse among those whose poor health status requires most attention. It is increasingly recognised by independent sources that the promotion of a healthy life style and the encouragement of community-and self-care require public action.(14) Such care is not cheap care and it is perhaps best not to leave health promotion entirely to private or even voluntary organisations which may have interests besides those of clients' health status.(15) Thus this care is not only expensive and not only requires state activity but it also is difficult to implement if people are not motivated or if it does not square with their own perceptions. Health education and promotion remain problematic.

Indeed, this is one of the four policy matters that our empirical material addresses. We saw particularly with respect to smoking, exercise and diet, how people may not share the opinions of medical experts. But their smoking, lack of exercise and so on are rational in terms of their own definitions and lives. It may be unlikely that exhortation will persuade all or most of those pursuing unhealthy styles of living to change their ways. This is not to argue against trying to stop people smoking and so on. We merely point to the difficulty. Secondly, we saw how some people define away serious, chronic conditions and regard themselves as healthy because of the need to continue working, looking after families and so on. While we do not know if the same people would have felt the need to continue to the detriment of their health in less pessimistic and less competitive times, it is a sad indictment of society that such should be the case. Thirdly, people saw health as embedded in quality of life and indeed life itself. Health is necessary to function adequately in British society while 'living in Britain' is seen as having serious consequences for health. Fourthly, there are differences in the ways in which people perceive and use health care facilities between places. Indeed, we may say that their perceptions affect the ways in which the facilities are used. A particular view may mean greater or less use. In any event, it means that the utilisation rates used in the formulae for allocating resources for health care to regions are further deficient. Not only, therefore, are they deficient in failing to incorporate morbidity or class indicators but there is also a more subtle effect in that use itself is shaped by perceptions of health, illness and the health care system.

What do these finding mean for policy? Together they suggest that policy, while recognising that resources are not infinite, must be sensitive to people's experiences. This may be best illustrated with respect to health education and promotion. It is possible to exhort people until the end of time but unless what is being exhorted fits with their experiences and needs they will not act upon it. Preventative and promotional health services must be context-relevant and their distribution should favour the most disadvantaged groups. It is partly a matter of presentation. Health education must be couched in a language accessible and understandable to its intended audience. People are not ignorant. We have been at pains to show that different groups act and think in different ways, all of which are rational in their own terms and in light of their needs and experiences.

Presentation is not only a matter for educational material. It also matters for the care facilities themselves. Many of the complaints about the health care system that we document stem from inadequate explanations of procedures by staff (clinical and clerical), medical attitudes towards patients and poor surroundings. There must be, therefore, a commitment to care and caring and to the well-being of individuals in the light of their particular circumstances. This commitment should not only be to care itself but to a particular set of care relations. As Deacon has pointed out,(16) the struggle for welfare is not just a matter of defending the interests of employees in state services but more one of transforming the relationships of welfare so that we are better able to care for each other. Finally, the findings suggest that care policies should be integrated so that health, welfare, housing and so on are functionally related with respect to provision. This is not to suggest that there is any easy way to integrate services. Bureaucratic loyalties and established practice conspire against change. Greater co-ordination of welfare services was suggested by the Royal Commission on the NHS.(17) Little has resulted. For over ten years, attempts have been made to initiate joint finance and planning between the health and personal social services.(18) It has had limited impact. But to say something is difficult is not to say that it is impossible. And it should be noted that many health problems are caused or exacerbated by low income, poor housing and so on. There may then be cost grounds for considering a more integrated approach to care provision. But on policy, our concluding remark must repeat our first: from our evidence, policy-making must resonate with the experiences of those that its implementation is meant to affect.

UNDERSTANDING AND EXPLANATION: COMMENTS ON METHOD

As a final task, however, we wish to leave consideration of policy and make some comments on method. In fact, we tried to make clear in the second chapter how the methodology we employed in this study works. That methodology allows the drawing of inferences so that understanding and explanation become possible. These goals of all science are based on a 'conceptual interference' with the data. In other words, the material derived from our respondents is set against theoretical concepts and ideas so as to enhance understanding. This is not a staged or sequential process of problem formulation, data collection, data analysis, explanation. In the terms used in chapter 2, the constructs of the second degree (scientific ones) derive from, relate to and inform those of the first degree (of everyday life) in a continuous process. The writing up of research can never adequately demonstrate this process. So that the reader has as clear a story line as possible to follow, presentation becomes stylised: the dynamic interplay of material and ideas (data and concepts) is played down, blind alleys which may have engaged the researcher for weeks or months and which seemed of seminal importance at the time are ignored and arguments which counter the main claims of the study may be 'suppressed'. The last named problem is of particular concern. It is extremely rare to discover a scientist who deliberately suppresses information because of its lack of fit. More likely is the case in which those individuals, events or stories which do not quite relate to the main lines of argument will be unconsciously underplayed. The only defence against such a difficulty is constant vigilance on the part of the researcher. She/he must also present her/his findings in such a way so that others could carry out a similar survey amongst the same or a similar population. Even then, we should not expect the same findings to be discovered. The second survey will not have been carried out by the same researcher or with the same respondents in that all of us are slightly different people as we meet new events and people. Readers can be useful in this process of checking too. Does the explanation seem right? Is it too pat? We must remember that life itself certainly is not. It is fuzzy, contradictory and seldom straightforward. We must also beware explanations that are so malleable that every case may be fitted to it. If it is that flexible, we should doubt its explanatory power for each and every individual case.

We have tried to make sense of how individuals make sense of their health and their social worlds in terms of the interpretative paradigm. We suggest that individuals construct their perceptions of health, illness and health care as well as their social worlds. These constructions take the form of meanings which people apply to various states, events and contexts. Although they take the form of 'subjective meanings', they are not just mental states independent of the material world. They are based on individual attributes and experiences and are thus derived from everyday life itself. This means, as we have tried to show, that a process of negotiation occurs in that individual characteristics such as class, ethnicity, disability are set against the demands of everyday life such as work, bringing up children, general functional capacity so that, on a specific level at least, the constructions and perceptions of health and illness are unique to the individual. Circumstances then shape perceptions but do not do so in any straightforward or mechanistic way. Some people regard a cold or mild influenza as reason enough to stay away from their place of paid employment. Others negotiate or so define away serious chronic conditions such as heart disease and diabetes and regard themselves as healthy so that they may carry out what they see as fundamentally important tasks. So it all depends. The social construction of the world - the basis for making sense of health and illness - depends on the type of person an individual is, her/his circumstances and attributes, her/his experiences and the demands placed on that individual by work, family and society.

These demands form the second element in our understanding of how people make sense. They do construct their social worlds but not in conditions of their own choosing. There are many constraints that act on people and 'force' them to behave and think in particular ways. We place force in inverted commas because coercion is seldom the major influence shaping people's lives. In the opening chapter, we outlined how a particular way of thinking can permeate the consciousness of all social groupings, although the ideas that it represents may not always be in the best or long-term interests of all. We highlighted the ideas of consumer capitalism. Elsewhere we have pointed to those of western medical culture. Both sets (and more) greatly influence the ways in which we think about life and what we would regard as possible or likely courses of action. In some circumstances - like those of our respondents - these ideas became manifest in a sense of pessimism, acquiescence and resignation.

These senses influence the ways in which individuals confront the most tangible constraints - institutions, structures, other people, events. Life in Britain was viewed almost universally in a pessimistic way. Quality of life and health were being adversely affected by events and forces over which individuals had little control. Work, money, unemployment, racism conspired to shape people's lives, health and perceptions of possibilities for life. Neighbourhood too had its effect, although some people regarded themselves as having greater control over that than the other forces. We must also remember that these forces do not operate independently of people's attributes, characteristics and constructions. They form the arena in which people make sense of the world, but they are also the world itself. What we need to make sense of is not somehow outside our lives but is a very real part of it. The wider environment, of which we are a part, is then a significant factor in shaping perceptions and behaviour.(19) The exact relationship between individual and environment and hence the shaping of beliefs and behaviour will again depend on circumstances. The structures that constrain our lives also enable us to respond in particular ways to events and crises.

The relationships between health perceptions and finance have been noted before, (20) as has the fatalistic or acquiescent response of certain people to particular illnesses.(21) This fatalism lends itself to the culture of poverty explanation, which suggests that as people experience poverty and the ensuing low status, a culture develops which has as its central features a sense of powerlessness, passivity and fatalism. People accept low levels of health, mis-trust modern medicine and are seldom future-oriented.(22) While we would not accept that the existence of a culture of poverty in Britain in the 1980s has been demonstrated, certain of the thesis's ideas seem useful. In chapter 4 we noted the circumstances that are shaping and helping to maintain a sense of resignation, fatalism and pessimism about the future among many of our working class respondents. These circumstances allow such feelings to flourish. They may continue to flourish in an increasingly low-wage, profit-oriented economy with increasingly inadequate state assistance to the needy.

We have deliberately broadened our interpretation again to the societal context so that our 'interference' with our data may be clearly perceived. This interference seems inevitable unless the words of our respondents are to remain disconnected sentences and stories. Their texts have to be read and interpreted. This view is well summarised by Geertz: "what the ethnographer is in fact faced with... is a multiplicity of complex conceptual structures, many of them superimposed upon or knotted into one another, which are at once strange, irregular, and inexplicit, and which he (sic) must contrive somehow first to grasp and then to render ... Doing ethnography is like trying to read (in the sense of 'constructing a reading of') a manuscript-foreign, faded, full of ellipses, incoherencies, suspicious emendations, and tendentious commentaries, but written not in conventionalised graphs of sound but in transient examples of shaded behaviour."(23) But the researcher's task does not end with this 'thick description'. It is necessary to interpret to understand and explain: "to draw large conclusions from small, but densely textured facts."(24)

But in such an approach, there remains a certain distance between the interpreter and the object of interpretation. People's accounts are engaged by the researcher as a reader rather than in the form of a dialogue,(25) although it is difficult to envision how a dialogue between researcher and people can be maintained except through a 'contract' that formalises withdrawal from the community and in terms of subjective interpretation as discussed in chapter 2. A different view of science is being put forward: one which rejects the idea of metanarratives and which uses poetry, art, film as well as oral accounts to help our understanding of the world.(26) In the words of Clifford, ethnography then "appears as writing, as collecting, as modernist collage, as imperial power, as subversive critique... a mode of travel, a way of understanding and getting around in a diverse world... One of the principal function of ethnography is "orientation".(27)

We accept that ethnographic research orients our understanding of the world. We also concur with the view that ethnographic truths are partial and committed and that their construction is an 'art' in the sense of a skilful fashioning of useful artifacts.(28) Further, if the use of artifacts other than oral accounts are meant to force us into recognising that our descriptions and explanations are interpretations relying on our classifications, orderings and conceptualisations, then they serve an important purpose. But beyond that, we remain uncertain as to the significance of following:

Because post-modern ethnography privileges 'discourse' over 'text', it foregrounds dialogue as opposed to monologue, and emphasises the cooperative and collaborative nature of the ethnographic situation in contrast to the ideology of the transcendental observer. In fact, it rejects the ideology of 'observer-observed', there being nothing observed and no one who is the observer. There is instead the mutual, dialogical production of a discourse, of a story of sorts.(29)

Does this mean that we are only participants and that we will all then produce a dialogical, partial and perhaps contradictory discourse with the role model being the community newspaper? This comment is not meant to belittle such endeavours in anthropology or the community newspaper. It is put forward from a concern as to the role of the ethnographer or scientist if we follow this route. On the one hand, it suggests that the only insights that matter are those from participants or insiders,(30) while on the other the partial and fragmentary nature of social understanding is best captured by journalists.(31) But we subscribe to the view that theoretical insight (see chapter 2), deriving from a specific socialisation, can add significantly to interpretation, understanding and explanation by providing the bases of conceptual interference. For all its partiality, incompleteness and evocation, an ethnographic account helps reconstruct reality.(32) It provides an outsider's view, albeit one sympathetic to insider accounts and one which tries to reduce the tensions between the inside and outside. This view is necessary for what Geertz called the large conclusions or the big picture. For us, the role of the scientist remains to understand and explain the nature of social reality. While others may, from their particular perspectives, also interpret the world, the ethnographer must make sense of how individuals make sense of their experiences and lives. And this we have tried to do in the context of health and illness in contemporary Britain.

FOOTNOTES

1. See J. Yates, _Why are we waiting? an analysis of hospital waiting lists_, Oxford UP, 1987.

2. J. Charlton, et al. Geographical variation in mortality from conditions amenable to medical intervention in England and Wales, _Lancet_ ii, 1983, 696.

3. This debate is reviewed in W.G. Runciman, _Relative deprivation and social justice_, RKP, 1966.

4. _ibid_ 27.

5. Deprivation and poverty are now increasingly seen as relative phenomena, i.e. relative to the standards, opportunities and styles treated as 'normal' in society. The critics of this view suggest that this is a nonsense as those without videos, holidays abroad and so on, will consider themselves poor. On this view too, poverty will never be abolished. Its constituent parts will merely change. The latter view must be accepted. In any society that makes a virtue out of competitive individualism and unequal distribution, relative deprivation will always exist. The ideas concerning relative (and absolute) deprivation are reviewed by J. Mack and S. Lansbury, _Poor Britain_, Allen and Unwin, 1985.

6. R. Jowell and C. Airey (eds.) _British social attitudes report_, Gower, 1985.

7. The characteristics of this set of values are now well established and analyzed. See, for example, D. Bull and P. Wilding (eds.) _Thatcherism and the poor_, CPAG, 1983; M. Loney, _The politics of greed_, Pluto Press, 1986.

8. M. Thatcher, _Let our children grow tall_, CPS, 1977, 97.

9. E. Durkheim, _Socialism and Saint Simon_, RKP, 1959, 200.

10. Loney _op cit._, 181.

11. See J. Eyles, _The geography of the national health_, Croom Helm, 1987, for an extended discussion.

12. DHSS, _Prevention and health_, DHSS, 1976, 102-3.

13. DHSS, _Care in action_, DHSS, 1981, Preface.

14. For a summary see A. Smith and B. Jacobson (eds.) _The nation's health_, Kings Fund, 1988.

15. These organisational and financial interests have been documented for the American context in N. Milio, The profitization of health promotion, _International Journal of Health Services_ 18, 1988, 573-85.

16. B. Deacon, <u>Social policy and socialism</u>, Pluto Press, 1983.

17. Great Britain, <u>Royal Commission on the NHS</u>, HMSO, 1979.

18. See A. Walker, <u>Social planning</u>, Blackwell, 1984.

19. The environment is seen as a real force because it has important consequences for people's lives. It is not an 'unnatural' force as Herzlich puts it. See C. Herzlich, <u>Health and Illness</u>, Academic Press, 1973.

20. For example, A Cartwright, <u>Human relations and hospital care</u>, RKP, 1964; J. Le Grand, <u>The strategy of equality</u>, Allen and Unwin, 1982.

21. This fatalism has been noted in the U.S. but not in some studies of the U.K. See, respectively, J. Rosenstock, Prevention of illness and maintenance of health, in J. Kosa and I.K. Zola (eds.) <u>Poverty and health</u>, Harvard UP, 1975; M. Blaxter and E. Patterson, <u>Mothers and daughters</u>, Heinemann, 1982.

22. The culture of poverty thesis was first developed by the American anthropologist, Oscar Lewis. See O. Lewis, <u>La vida</u>, Panther, 1968. It is critically reviewed in P. Townsend, <u>Poverty in the United Kingdom</u>, Penguin, 1979.

23. C. Geertz, <u>The interpretation of cultures</u>, Harper, 1973, 10.

24. <u>ibid</u>, 28.

25. See the discussion in G.E. Marcus and M.J.J. Fisher, <u>Anthropology as cultural critique</u>, University of Chicago Press, 1986.

26. See <u>ibid</u>, chapter 3 and J. Clifford, <u>The predicament of culture</u>, Harvard U.P., 1988.

27. <u>ibid</u>, 13.

28. See J. Clifford, Introduction: partial truths in J. Clifford and G.E. Marcus (eds.) <u>Writing culture</u>, University of California Press, 1986.

29. S.A. Tyler, Post-modern ethnography, in Clifford and Marcus <u>op. cit</u>. 126.

30. This seems like a replay of the arguments put forward by ethnomethodologists that respondents alone know their own life histories, the cultural contexts of which they are part, and their own self-concepts and practical purposes within the interview. It is the respondent then who decides what to say and the precise meaning and significance of what she/he is saying. See A.V. Cicourel, <u>Cognitive sociology</u>, Free Press, 1974.

31. This is not to say that journalists have not produced excellent accounts of the social world, usually with commentary as in Seabrook's work but sometimes without, just allowing people to speak for themselves. See J. Seabrook, _Unemployment_, Paladin, 1982. As an example of the latter, T. Parker, _The people of providence_, Penguin, 1984.

32. The phrase is taken from Schwartz and Jacobs, who see qualitative sociology as being in the reality reconstruction business, learning to see the world as our respondents see it and then ordering and interpreting it by using scientific constructs. See H. Schwartz and J. Jacobs, _Qualitative sociology_, Free Press, 1979 and chapter 2 above.

Bibliography

Abel-Smith B. and Townsend, P., (1965), <u>The Poor and the Poorest</u>, Bell.

Abrams, P., (1977), 'Community Care', <u>Policy and Politics</u>, vol. 6, 125-51.

Allsop, J., (1984), <u>Health Policy and the NHS</u>, Longman.

Alt, J., (1976), Beyond Class, <u>Telos</u>, 28, 55-80.

Bauman, Z., (1982), <u>Memories of Class</u>, RKP.

Berger, P. and Luckmann, T., (1967), <u>The Social Construction of Reality</u>, Penguin.

Bhaskar, R., <u>The Possibility of Naturalism</u>, Harvester.

Blackwell, T. and Seabrook, J., (1985), <u>A World Still to Win</u>, Faber and Faber.

Blaxter, M., (1983), 'The causes of disease', <u>Social Science and Medicine</u>, 17, 59-69.

Blaxter, M., (1985), 'Self-definition of Health Status and Consulting Rates in Primary Care', <u>Quarterly Journal of Social Affairs</u>, vol. 1, 131-71.

Blaxter, M. and Patterson, E., (1982), <u>Mothers and Daughters</u>, Heinemann.

Blumhagen, D.W., (1980), 'Hypertension', <u>Culture, Medicine and Psychiatry</u>, vol. 4, 197-227.

Boggs, C., (1976), <u>Gramsci's Maxism</u>, Pluto Press.

Brook, R. and Ware, J.E., (1979), 'Overview of Adult Health Status Measures', <u>Medical Care</u>, (Supplement) vol. 17(7), 1-31.

Brotherson, J., (1976), 'Inequality: Is It Inevitable?' in Carter, C.O. and Peel, J. (eds.) <u>Equalities and Inequalities in Health</u>, Academic Press.

Brown, C., (1984), <u>Black and White Britain</u>, Heinemann.

Burgess, R., (1984), <u>In the Field</u>, Allen and Unwin.

Burgess, R., (ed.) (1982), <u>Field Research</u>, Allen and Unwin.

Butler, J.R. and Vaile, M., (1984), <u>Health and Health</u>

Services, RKP.

Calnan, M., (1984), 'Clinical Uncertainty', Sociology of Health and Illness, vol. 6, 74-85.

Calnan, M., (1987), Health and Illness, Tavistock.

Calnan, M., (1988), 'Lay Evaluation of Medicine and Medical Practice', International Journal of Health Services, vol. 18, 311-22.

Carstairs, V. and Patterson, P.E., (1966), 'Distribution of Hospital Patients by Social Class', Health Bulletin 24, 59-65.

Cartwright, A., (1964), Human Relations and Hospital Care, RKP.

Cartwright, A., (1967), Patients and Their Doctors, RKP.

Cartwright, A. and Anderson, R., (1981), General Practice Revisited, Tavistock.

Central Statistical Office, (1985), Social Trends, 15.

Central Statistical Office, (1986), Social Trends, 16.

Central Statistical Office, (1988), Social Trends, 18.

Charlton, J. et al., (1983), 'Geographical Variation in Mortality from Conditions Amenable to Medical Intervention in England and Wales', Lancet, vol. ii, 691-6.

Cicourel, A.V., (1974), Cognitive Sociology, Free Press.

Clifford, J., (1986), 'Introduction: Partial Truths', in J. Clifford and G.E. Marcus (eds.), Writing Culture, University of California Press.

Clifford, J., (1988), The Predicament of Culture, Harvard University Press.

Coates, E. and Silburn, (1970), Poverty: the Forgotten Englishmen, Penguin.

Collins, E. and Klein, R., (1980), 'Equality and the NHS', British Medical Journal, vol. 281, 111-5.

Cornwell, J., (1984), Hard-earned Lives, Tavistock.

Cowie, B., (1976), 'The Cardiac Patient's Perception of his Heart Attack', Social Science and Medicine, vol. 10, 87-96.

Cox, C. and Mead, A., (eds.), (1974), A Sociology of Medical Practice, Collier-Macmillan.

Deacon, B., (1983), Social Policy and Socialism, Pluto Press.

Department of the Environment, (1984), English Housing Condition Survey 1981, DOE.

Department of Health and Social Security, (1976), Prevention and Health, DHSS.

Department of Health and Social Security, (1980), Inequalities in Health, DHSS.

Department of Health and Social Security, (1981), Care in Action, DHSS.

Department of Health and Social Security, (1988), Review of the RAWP Formula, DHSS.

Dingwall, R., (1976), Aspects of Illness, Martin Robertson.

Donovan, J., (1984), 'Ethnicity and Health' Social Science and Medicine, vol. 19, 663-70.

Donovan, J., (1986), We Don't Buy Sickness, It Just Comes, Gower.

Doyal, L., (1979), The Political Economy of Health, Pluto Press.

Durkheim, E., (1959), Socialism and Saint Simon, RKP.

Eisenberg, L. and Kleinman, A. (eds.), (1981), The Relevance of Social Science for Medicine, D. Reidel.

Eyles, J., (1979), Area-based Policies for the Inner City, in Herbert D. and Smith, D.M. (eds.), Social Problems and the City, Oxford UP.

Eyles, J., (1985), Senses of Place, Silverbrook Press.

Eyles, J., (1987), The Geography of the National Health, Croom Helm.

Eyles, J. and Donovan, J., (1986a) Regional Variations in Perceptions and Experiences of Health and Health Care, End of Research Report, ESRC (Grant no. G 00232140).

Eyles, J. and Donovan, J., (1986b), 'Making Sense of Sickness and Care', Transactions, Institute of British Geographers, vol. 11, 415-27.

Eyles, J. and Woods, K.J., (1983), The Social Geography of Medicine and Health, St. Martin's Press.

Eyles, J. and Woods, K.J., (1986), 'Who Cares What Care', Social Science and Medicine, vol. 23, 1087-92.

Fitzpatrick, R., (1984), The Experience of Illness, Tavistock.

Fothergill, S. and Vincent, J., (1985), The State of the Nation, Pan.

Freidson, E., (1970), Profession of Dominance, Dodd Mead.

Gaines, A.D., (1979), 'Definition and Diagnoses', Culture, Medicine and Psychiatry, vol. 3, 381-418.

Gamble, A. and Walton, P.,(1976), Capitalism and Crises, Macmillan.

Garrity, T., (1981), 'Medical Compliance', Social Science and Medicine, vol. 15E, 215-22.

Geertz, C., (1973), The Interpretation of Cultures, Harper.

Giddens, A., (1976), New Rules of Sociological Method, Hutchinson.

Giddens, A., (1984), The Constitution of Society, Polity Press.

Goldthorpe, J. et al., (1969), The Affluent Worker in the Class Structure, Cambridge University Press.

Great Britain, (1979), Royal Commission on the NHS, HMSO.

Hall, S., (1984), 'The Culture Gap', Marxism Today, vol. 28(1), 18-22.

Hammersley, M. and Atkinson, M., (1983), Ethnography, Tavistock.

Health Education Council, (1987), The Health Divide, HEC.

Heller, A., (1983), A Theory of History, RKP.

Heller, A., (1984), Everyday Life, RKP.

H.M. Treasury, (1986), Government Expenditure Plans, HMSO.

Herzlich, C., (1983), Health and Illness, Academic Press.

Hindess, B., (1977), Philosophy and the Social Sciences, Harvester.

Horowitz, A, (1978), 'Family, Kin and Friend Networks in Psychiatric Help-Seeking, Social Science and Medicine, vol. 12, 297-304.

Hunt, S. and McEwen, J., (1980), 'The Development of a Subjective Health Indicator', Sociology of Health and Illness, vol. 2, 231-6.

Hunt, S. et al., (1981), 'The Nottingham Health Profile', Social Science and Medicine, vol. 15A, 221-9.
Hunt, S. et al., (1986), Measuring Health Status, Croom Helm.

Ignu, U., (1979), 'Stages in Health Seeking', Social Science and Medicine, vol. 13A, 445-56.
Illich, I., (1977), Limits to Medicine, Penguin.

Jowell, R. and Airey, C., (eds.), (1985), British Social Attitudes: the 1984 Report, Gower.
Jowell, R. et al., (eds.), (1988), British Social Attitudes: the Fifth Report, Gower.

Le Grand, J., (1982), The Strategy of Equality, Allen and Unwin.
Lewis, O., (1968), La Vida, Panther.
Littlewood, R. and Lipsedge, M. (1982), Aliens and Alienists, Penguin.
Lock, M., (1982), 'Models and Practice in Medicine', Culture, Medicine and Psychiatry, vol. 6, 261-80.
Loney, M., (1986), The Politics of Greed, Pluto Press.

Mack, J. and Lansbury, S. (1985), Poor Britain, Allen and Unwin.
Manwaring, T. and Sigler, N., (eds.), (1985), Breaking the Nation, Pluto Press.
Marcus, G.E. and Fisher, M.M., (1986), Anthropology as Cultural Critique, University of Chicago Press.
Marmot, M.G., (1986), 'Mortality Decline and Widening Social Inequalities', Lancet, vol. ii, 274-6.
Marwick, A., (1980), Class: Image and Reality, Fontana.
Marwick, A., (1982), British Society Since 1945, Penguin.
McKinlay, J. (1981), 'Social Network Influences on Morbid Episodes and the Career of Help Seeking', in Eisenberg and Kleinman op. cit.
Mechanic, D., (1978), Medical Sociology, Free Press.
Mehan, H., (1979), Learning Lessons: Social Organisation in the Classroom, Harvard University Press.
Milio, N., (1988), 'The Profitization of Health Promotion', International Journal of Health Services, vol. 18, 573-85.
Mishra, R., (1984), The Welfare State in Crisis, Wheatsheaf.
Mitchell, J.C. (1983), 'Case and Situation Analysis, Sociological Review, vol. 31, 187-211.

Navarro, V., (1974), Medicine Under Capitalism, Prodist.
Noyce, J. et al., (1975), 'Regional Variations in the Allocation of Financial Resources to Community Health Services', Lancet 1, 345-7.

Office of Health Economics, (1984), Compendium of Health Statistics, (5th Edition), OHE.
Office of Population Censuses and Surveys, (1984a) The General Household Survey, HMSO.
OPCS, (1984b), Ward Monitor: West Midlands, HMSO.
OPCS, (1984c), Ward Monitor: Greater London, HMSO.
OPCS (1984d), Ward Monitor: West Yorkshire, HMSO.

Parker, T., (1984), The People of Providence, Penguin.

Parsons, T., (1951), The Social System, Free Press.

Pill, R. and Stott, N.C.H., (1982), 'Concepts of Illness Causation and Responsibility', Social Science and Medicine, vol. 16, 43-52.

Rathwell, T. and Phillips, D., (eds.), (1986), Health, Race and Ethnicity, Croom Helm.

Reid, I., (1981), Social Class Differences in Britain, Grant McIntyre.

Rickard, J.E. , (1976), 'Per Capita Expenditure of English Area Health Authorities', British Medical Journal, vol. 277, 299-300.

Roberts, H., (1985), Patient Patients, Pandora Press.

Rosenstock, J, (1975), 'Prevention of Illness and Maintenance of Health', in Kosa, J. and Zola, I.K. (eds.), Poverty and Health, Harvard UP.

Runciman, W.G., (1966), Relative Deprivation and Social Justice, RKP.

Rutter, M. and Nadge, N., (1976), Cycles of Disadvantage, Heinemann.

Salloway, J. and Dillon, P., (1973), 'A Comparison of Family Networks and Friend Networks in Health Care Utilisation', Journal of Comparative Family Studies, vol. 4, 131-42.

Schutz, A., (1962), Collected Papers, vol. 1, Nijhoff.

Schwartz, H. and Jacobs, J., (1979), Qualitative Sociology, Free Press.

Scrambler, A., (1981), 'Kinship and Friendship Networks and Women's Demands for Primary Care', Journal of the Royal College of General Practitioners, vol. 26, 746-50.

Seabrook, J., (1982), Unemployment, Paldin.

Sheiham, H. and Quick, A., (1982), The Rickets Report, Harringey CHC and CRC.

Silverman, D., (1985), Qualitative Methodology and Sociology, Gower.

Simon, R., (1982), Gramsci's Political Thought, Lawrence and Wishart.

Smith, A. and Jacobson, B., (eds.), (1988), The Nation's Health, Kings Fund.

Stevenson, I.N., (1980), 'Editorial Comment', Social Science and Medicine, vol. 14B,1.

Suchman, E.A., (1964), 'Socio-medical Variations Among Ethnic Groups', American Journal of Sociology, 70, 319-31.

Thatcher, M., (1977), Let Our Children Grown Tall, CPS.

Todd, J., (1985), 'Cruel Absurdity of Telling Your Patients Everything', Doctor, vol. 15, 37.

Toland, S., (1980), 'Changes in Living Standards Since the 1950s', Social Trends, vol. 10, 13-38.

Townsend, P., (1979), Poverty in the United Kingdom, Penguin.

Townsend, P. and Davidson, D., (1982), Inequalities in Health, Penguin.

Tuckett, D.A. et al., (1986), Meetings between Experts, Tavistock.

Tyler, S.A., (1986), 'Post-modern ethnography' in Clifford,

J. and Marcus, G.E. (eds.) Writing Culture, University of California Press.

Urry, J., (1981), The Anatomy of Capitalist Societies, Macmillan.

Voysey, M., (1975), A Constant Burden, RKP.

Walker, A., (1984), Social Planning, Blackwell.
Walters, V., (1980), Class Inequality and Health Care, Croom Helm.
Ware, J.E., (1978), 'The Effects of Acquiescent Response Set', Medical Care, 16, 327-36.
Westergaard, J.and Resler, H., (1975), Class in A Capitalist Society, Penguin.
Wildavsky, A., (1980), The Art and Craft of Policy Analysis, Macmillan.
Williams, R., (1983), 'Concepts of Health' Sociology, 17, 185-205.
Wolff, K., (1978), 'Phenomenology and Sociology', in Bottomore, T., and Nisbett, R. (eds.), A History of Sociological Analysis, Heinemann.

Yates, J., (1987), Why Are We Waiting? An Analysis of Hospital Waiting Lists, Oxford UP.

Zola, I.K., (1972), 'Medicine as an Institution of Social Control', Sociological Review, vol. 21, 615-30.